Restorative Techniques in Paediatric Dentistry

Clinical Techniques in Dentistry

Restorative Techniques in Paediatric Dentistry

An Illustrated Guide to the Restoration of Extensively Carious Primary Teeth

Monty S Duggal BDS, MDS, FDSRCS
Martin E J Curzon BDS, MSc, PhD, FRCD(C), FDSRCS
Stephen A Fayle BDS, MDSc, MRCD(C), FDSRCS
Maxine A Pollard BDS, MDSc, PhD, MRCD(C)
Angus J Robertson AIMI, RMIP

with contributions from

Elizabeth A O'Sullivan BChD, MDentSci, MRCD(C)
K Jack Toumba BSc(Hons), MSc, BChD

Paediatric Dentistry, Division of Child Dental Health
Leeds Dental Institute, University of Leeds, Leeds, England

Colour photography by **Angus J Robertson**

MARTIN DUNITZ

© **Martin Dunitz Ltd** 1995

First published in the United Kingdom in 1995 by Martin Dunitz Ltd, The Livery House, 7–9 Pratt Street, London NW1 OAE

ISBN 1-85317-197-2

A CIP catalogue record of this title is available from the British Library.

Composition by Scribe Design, Gillingham, Kent, UK
Colour origination by Imago Publishing Ltd
Printed and bound in Singapore by Kyodo Printing Co (S'pore) Pte Ltd

Contents

Foreword

Clinical paediatric dentistry is a demanding subject. This book by Professor Martin E. J. Curzon and colleagues concentrates on a very important issue in the clinical treatment of children — the rational restoration of extensively carious primary teeth. Despite effective preventive programmes, which have resulted in a tremendous improvement in the oral health of children and adolescents, in any population there will always be a group of children with a high caries activity resulting in extensive carious lesions. The successful treatment of such children, especially with regard to primary dentition, is a very difficult and complicated task. A golden rule in the treatment strategy for this group is to perform all clinical procedures to such a high standard that retreatment is unnecessary and no further work should be needed on the tooth before normal exfoliation.

This philosophy is the backbone of this book, which presents a detailed step-by-step guide to help the reader reach the required level of excellence for the treatment of extensively carious primary teeth. Using first-class photographic material, all the important procedures are described in an impressive and instructive way, and useful comments on the scientific background and prognosis are provided. There are detailed chapters on treatment planning, local analgesia, rubber dam technique, pulp therapy for primary teeth, stainless steel crowns and strip crowns for primary incisors. This information is consolidated in the last chapter by means of a number of case reports.

The authors are to be congratulated on an excellent book that should be read and reread by all those aiming to perform high-quality paediatric dentistry, which is cost-effective both for the dentist and the patient and has long-term preventive implications. I warmly recommend this book and believe that it will be well accepted by the dental profession.

Göran Koch
Odont dr., Professor
Chairman Pediatric Dentistry
The Institute for Postgraduate Dental Education
Jönköping, Sweden

Dedicated to Megan Fayle

Preface

Although there has been a decline in dental caries in recent years, a significant number of children in the United Kingdom and in many other countries still have the disease. It is essential that their teeth be restored as quickly and efficiently as possible and to the highest standard.

Restorations in primary teeth should last until such time as the teeth are exfoliated. If they are placed correctly, they should never need repairing or replacing.

A new system of payment for dentistry for children, 'capitation', has been introduced in the United Kingdom. Under this system, dentists are remunerated with a yearly standard fee, which provides for the total dental care of a child, no matter what dental care is required. Although this has been most widely introduced in the United Kingdom, capitation systems have been used in other countries as well. If such a scheme is to be financially successful for the dentist, he or she must implement an excellent prevention programme, and any restorations must be of the highest quality.

The economics of repeated restoration of the same teeth is not remunerative. Therefore the dentist either cannot afford to treat the child or takes the approach of 'supervised neglect'. The result of this is that confidence in the dentist's ability to care for the child declines, and both the child's and the parents' tolerance and acceptance of further care are affected.

We have therefore produced this atlas of restorative techniques for primary molars and incisors to aid dentists and students in the provision of high-quality restorations for the primary dentition. Our intention has been to describe a detailed step-by-step procedure for treating carious teeth. In using an atlas format, we hope that each step will be clear and that students and dentists will be able to undertake all of these types of restorations.

We have restricted ourselves to the description of the techniques of pulp therapy, stainless steel crowns and strip crowns. We have deliberately not included restorations using amalgam, composite resin or glass ionomer cements. This is because the use of amalgam and composite resin for one- and two-surface restorations in primary teeth has been described extensively in many other books. We feel that glass ionomer cements are of limited use for broken down primary teeth, and should be used only as temporary restorations.

There are no contraindications to the restoration of primary teeth, with the exception of the very young (under 3 years of age), mentally compromised and certain children with medical complications, local analgesia, rubber dam. All restorations illustrated in this atlas are possible and desirable in dental practice. The cooperation of the child is obviously necessary, and this needs to be gained before restorative treatment is started.

The approach taken is to describe each technique with the minimum amount of text and to illustrate it with photographs. This step-by-step approach shows each facet of restoring a primary tooth.

The cases have all been taken from the records of children treated in our clinic at Leeds by undergraduates, postgraduates or members of staff in paediatric dentistry. The children all required extensive dental care, but were initially reasonably cooperative and their behaviour management was part of the care given, although not described here. Obviously, to complete the type of restorations illustrated, good cooperation was required.

The restorations shown here should be well within the capability of any dentist with an interest in the dental care of children. No special skills are required nor need the type of work be performed only by specialist paediatric dentists.

In our opinion, every child with dental caries deserves the standard of care shown in this atlas.

MSD MEJC
MAP SAF AJR

Acknowledgements

The preparation of an atlas such as this has involved many of our colleagues and postgraduate students. Some of the illustrations used here have been gleaned from the presentation cases of our postgraduates as part of their masters degree examinations, from undergraduate treatment cases and from our own patients.

We are particularly grateful to our colleagues who have helped with the preparation of the illustrations and text. Our postgraduate students were very understanding when we photographed procedures while they were treating their patients. Inevitably this slowed up the treatment.

Over the past few years, we have been indebted to the members of the Medical and Dental Illustration Department at Leeds who have taken many pictures of our patients for teaching purposes. Some of this material has also been included here. We would like to acknowledge David Hawkridge and Mary Lunn for their excellent photography, Joyce Hindmarsh for duplicating all of the radiographs used here, and also Anna Durbin for illustrations (Figures 1.6 and 1.9). We are particularly indebted to Alison Campbell of our publishers, Martin Dunitz, for her patience and encouragement in the preparation of this atlas.

Finance from 3M Health Care Ltd was given to support additional photography, and for the transfer of clinical slide material into good quality prints for the illustrations.

Treatment Planning

I

Children as individuals

A treatment plan must be developed and designed to provide high-quality restorative care for each individual child's needs. The details will vary according to the types of restorations needed, as will the sequence of placing restorations.

In this book the objective is to provide an atlas describing the techniques for the *restorative* care of children, and therefore the approach to treatment planning is very much orientated to that end. It is accepted that every child will require some degree of preventive dentistry and behaviour management, but these subjects will not be covered here.

Philosophy of treatment planning

In planning for the restoration of teeth, allowance must be made for two types of children. The first will be those for whom no restorative care has been attempted in the past, but who now do need it. For these children a sequenced introduction to the procedures of restoring teeth is needed. Treatment planning for them must include a step-by-step introduction to the use of pain control (local analgesia), use of rotary instruments, rubber dam and the placing of restorations. The time needed for this introduction may be anything from a few minutes to several visits.

Most children will not normally be afraid, and one of the important aspects of providing care for them will be to ensure that they do not develop a fear of dentistry.

The second group of children comprises those who may already have had some restorations or perhaps attempted restorations. With these children there may be a history of being totally uncooperative or only reluctant to cooperate but persuadable. In such cases the treatment planning must take into account the degree of coopera-

tion and again an amount of time allowed for behaviour modification.

In this atlas it is assumed that a child is cooperative or that cooperation has been obtained.

The technique of treatment planning is to obtain all the necessary information on the dental history and dental status of a child. Using this information, a plan of dental visits is drawn up so as to complete the restorative care needed in the shortest possible time appropriate for that child. It is our philosophy that the ideal approach for restoring children's teeth involves the practice of quadrant dentistry.

Diagnosis

The dental problems of a child must be assessed before a treatment plan is designed. This involves not only examining the teeth but also assessing the child's behaviour. This should start before the child has entered the dental office and should begin by observing the child with his or her parents or carers in the waiting room. As the family enter, the child's behaviour and relationship with parents or carers should be observed. It is at this stage that any apprehension or difficult behaviour should be noted, since it will affect the sequence of restorative procedures and hence the treatment plan.

A history should be taken from the parents, including details of previous behaviour, restorations or attempted restorations. In addition, the parents should be asked if previous restorative work has been with or without local analgesia and rubber dam. Any previous history of extractions, again with either local analgesia or general anaesthesia, should be noted. These details should be recorded on a dental history form (Figure 1.1).

The first visit will include a simple examination of the dentition, with an assessment of the extent of dental caries, oral hygiene, gingivitis and periodontal disease. All oral tissues should be

> Likes to be called ....

DENTAL HISTORY

Name.. Date of birth ....

Address.. Siblings   1. .... Age ....

....   2. .... Age ....

....   3. .... Age ....

Medical history:...

....

....

....

Past dental history: Check-ups   Yes__   No__   Extractions   Yes__   No__

                      Fillings   Yes__   No__   L.A.   Yes__   No__

                      Fiss. Seal. Yes__   No_   G.A.   Yes__   No__

Liked:...

Disliked:...

Parents' assessment of previous behaviour: Excellent. Good. Fair. Poor. Bad.

Parents' assessment of expected behaviour: Good. Cooperative. Resistant.

EXTRA-ORAL EXAMINATION

....

....

INTRA-ORAL EXAMINATION

....

....

....

DENTAL CHARTING:

R	17	16	5	4	3	2	1	1	2	3	4	5	26	27	L
	47	46	5	4	3	2	1	1	2	3	4	5	36	37	

DIAGNOSIS

....

....

....

Figure 1.1 Dental history form.

examined for health and possible pathology. Before restorative care is started, the oral hygiene should be of a good standard, and the child's behaviour should have been assessed and measures taken to ensure cooperation.

Dental caries assessment

For the restoration of primary and young adult teeth, the extent of dental caries must be known. A clinical examination with a dental mirror and good lighting is required, with a dry field. The presence of all carious lesions and restorations must be recorded on a suitable dental chart. If available, transillumination is also helpful.

In particular, the following should be noted about the dental caries in each tooth:

- staining of pits and fissures;
- discolouration of the enamel;
- condition of the marginal ridge, whether intact or broken (Figure 1.2).

At the same time, the presence of chronic or acute abscesses should be noted, as well as drain-ing sinuses, which would indicate pulpal pathology (Figure 1.3).

Existing restorations should be examined with care for recurrent caries and for the type and integrity of the restorations. In particular, glass ionomer cements and composite resin restorations should be examined most critically, since their success rates in primary teeth are poor and they often need replacement. An example of a poor quality glass ionomer restoration in a primary molar that has failed is shown in Figure 1.4. Too often, an attempt is made to restore a large cavity in a primary tooth with a material that will not hold for very long. Leakage around the margins or breakdown of the margins leads to failure of the restoration. In many cases the cavity was originally quite deep, and irreversible pulpal necrosis occurs when the tooth dies and an abscess ensues. This is the situation illustrated in Figure 1.4.

Attention should also be paid to the state of the primary incisors. When nursing bottle caries has occurred, an assessment of the possibility of restoring these teeth should be made. In most cases even quite badly broken teeth can be restored with strip crowns, as long as there is sufficient coronal dentine and enamel left. Even four badly decayed maxillary incisors (Figure 1.5) can be retained.

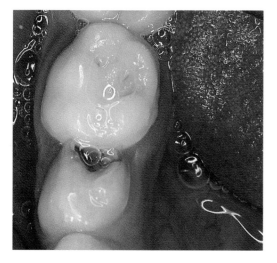

Figure 1.2 Photograph of primary molars showing broken marginal ridge. Where over one-third of the marginal ridge has been lost, pulpal involvement has occurred and pulp treatment (pulpotomy or pulpectomy) should be planned (see Chapter 4).

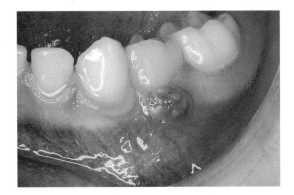

Figure 1.3 Photograph of primary molars showing a draining sinus on a first primary molar with a failed glass ionomer restoration. This tooth must be treated with a pulpectomy (see Chapter 4).

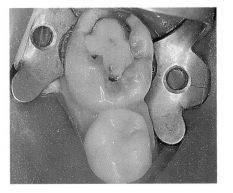

Figure 1.4 Photograph of a primary molar with a failed glass ionomer cement restoration, now requiring pulp treatment and a preformed metal crown (see Chapters 4 and 5).

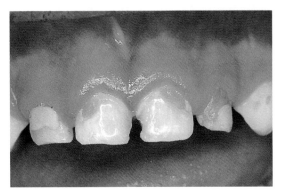

Figure 1.5 Photograph showing decayed primary maxillary incisors due to nursing bottle caries. These can be restored with strip crowns (see Chapter 6).

Dental charting

The condition of all teeth should be recorded on a suitable chart. It is important that all teeth, existing restorations (of no matter what quality) and sites of dental caries must be charted. The presence of sound restorations should also be recorded (usually in blue or black) as should all dental caries (in red).

Any stained, discoloured or broken marginal ridges, stained pits and fissures, abscesses or sinuses should also be noted, on the chart. Fractured teeth (incisors) should be recorded, although their restoration is not dealt with in this book.

Accurate dental records for dental caries and restorations are needed prior to drawing up a treatment plan, but are also essential for medicolegal requirements. A complete charting should also be completed at each recall visit when a new course of care is planned. This should be done even if no new restorative procedures are indicated.

An intra-oral charting together with diagnostic quality radiographs and other diagnostic tests enable a logical treatment plan to be drawn up.

The details of the treatment plan, with an outline of the number of treatment visits, should be discussed with the child's parents. This is essential, because the success of the treatment will be dependent on parental enthusiasm and support. If a parent is not willing to bring the child, or cannot afford the necessary costs in time and money, then an alternative plan will need to be drawn up. However, for our purposes we have assumed that all treatment is accepted by the parent or carer, and restorative work can be completed with the cooperation of parent and child.

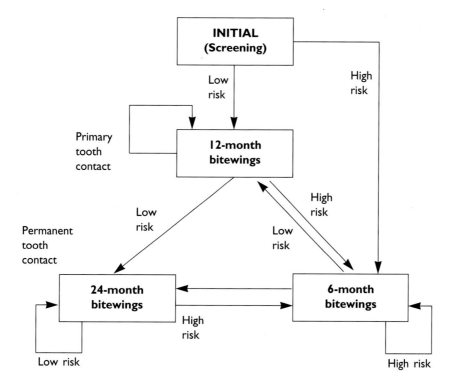

Figure 1.6 Scheme for deciding when to take bitewing radiographs of a child based upon dental caries experience.

It is recommended that once a treatment plan has been agreed with the parent that it be signed by him or her. This is particularly important when financial payment is involved.

Radiographs

It is necessary to repeat radiographs for dental caries diagnosis at intervals. This will depend on the caries history of the child. There are no hard and fast rules regarding the intervals for the taking of bitewing radiographs, but one suggested scheme is shown in Figure 1.6. This is based upon the past caries history of a child and indicates whether bitewings are needed at 6- or 12-month intervals for the primary dentition. As the caries history of a child develops, it becomes necessary to reassess the need for radiographs at each recall examination. If a child does not develop new caries lesions then the interval between taking bitewing radiographs should be increased.

A good approach requires two recall examinations without new carious lesions before this is done.

After one year (two recalls) without new lesions, the bitewing interval is increased to one year. After a further year without any evidence of dental caries, the interval is increased to 18 months. However, if at any time new caries is diagnosed or there is caries around restorations then the interval between bitewing radiographs is returned to six months.

This approach is used not only for the primary dentition but also for the mixed and permanent dentitions, as indicated in Figure 1.6.

The set of radiographs taken for a child at any one course of dental care will vary according to the needs and age of the child. At least one orthopantomogram or its equivalent should be available at least once during the development stage of the dentition (age 6 years). Bitewings and/or peri-apical views are also appropriate. Two suggested sequences of radiographs are shown in Figures 1.7 and 1.8.

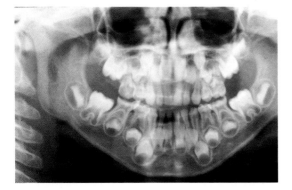

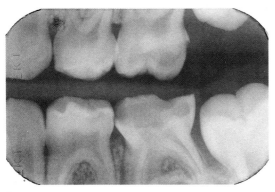

L

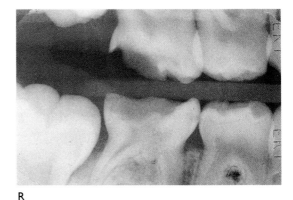

R

Figure 1.7 A typical sequence of radiographs for a preschool child, comprising an orthopantomogram and a set of bitewings. These views are designed to show all alveolar bone structures, development of primary and secondary teeth, and peri-apical or furcation pathology associated with the primary teeth and bone and other structures of the maxilla and mandible. Bitewings show the presence/absence of dental caries.

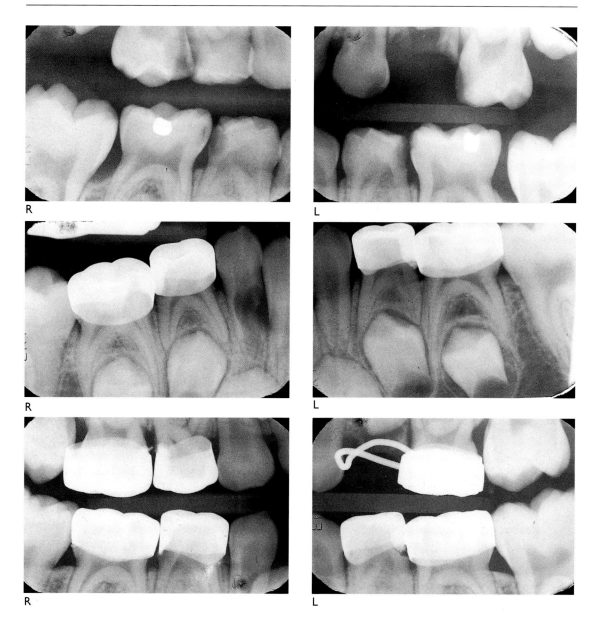

Figure 1.8 A suggested sequence of radiographs for a child of school age who has already had a number of restorative procedures. The bitewings serve to diagnose new or recurrent caries, while the peri-apical views are usually taken of the primary molars for pathology secondary to pulp therapy.

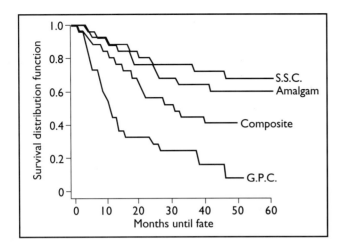

Figure 1.9 Survival rate of various types of restorations in primary teeth over a period of five years. Restorations were placed by staff and students in a dental school paediatric dental clinic. SSC, preformed metal crown; amalgam, amalgam restoration; composite, composite resin; GPC, glass ionomer cement.

Choice of restoration

The type of restoration used for a primary tooth will depend on:

- the tooth to be restored;
- past caries history;
- child cooperation.

An important consideration in restoring primary teeth, as with all teeth, is that a tooth should only need restoring once. A need for repeated restoration of a primary tooth indicates bad dental care. The cooperation of a child may well deteriorate if for every course of treatment the same teeth need restoration. It will also not encourage confidence on the part of the parent if teeth have to be restored repeatedly.

Various research groups have studied the longevity or failure rate of restorations of primary teeth. Our own work on this (Figure 1.9) has shown that where there has been caries on at least two surfaces or a marginal ridge has broken, the preformed metal crown (stainless steel crown) is the restoration of choice. Amalgam at present is a valuable restorative material in the primary dentition, and is indicated for one-surface or small two-surface restorations.

It is clear from Figure 1.9 that composite resin restorations and glass ionomer cements under clinical conditions did not survive beyond 48 months (four years) out of the possible five years

covered by the study. Other researchers have found similar results. On this basis, our present recommendation is that great care must be taken when composite resins and glass ionomer cements are used for primary molars.

Both composite resins and glass ionomer cements are technique-sensitive, and ideally need to be placed under rubber dam. Therefore these types of restorations are recommended for small single surfaces only. Glass ionomer cements can be used as semi-permanent restorations in primary molars when the teeth are close to exfoliation. Alternatively, glass ionomer cements may be used as a temporary measure for a few months until a permanent restoration can be placed.

Local analgesia

It is our philosophy that local analgesia should be routinely used in the restoration of primary teeth. In a cooperative child there are no contraindications for its use other than very young age (below approximately 2½ years). There is also no contraindication to the use of a mandibular block in children, although we advocate the use of the 'rule of 10' to determine whether a block or an infiltration is used for primary mandibular molars. This approach takes the age of the child plus the number of the tooth (canine = 3, first molar = 4, second molar = 5). If this is more than 10 then a mandibular block is needed. If it is less than 10 then an infiltration is appropriate. Thus if a restoration is required in a second molar in a 3-year-old, (5 + 3 = 8) then an infiltration is indicated.

We strongly advocate the use of topical analgesia with a flavoured benzocaine cream. A number of flavours (mint, cherry, bubblegum etc.) are available and have the advantage that they enable the child to have a choice, and therefore a degree of participation, in restoring their teeth. This can be very important as part of the behaviour management of the child.

A short-acting analgesic should be used, such as prilocaine, which provides a sufficient duration of analgesia (30–45 minutes) to accomplish the necessary restorations in a quadrant. At the same time, the soft tissue analgesia should be wearing off by the time the child leaves the dental office.

The use of local analgesia in children is described more fully in Chapter 2.

Rubber dam

Rubber dam is the technique most widely advocated in dental teaching—yet the most widely neglected in dental practice. However, we believe that the restoration of primary teeth should always, as far as possible, be carried out under rubber dam. It is essential for pulp therapy, and highly desirable if quadrant dentistry is to be accomplished.

Order of restorations

It is important to start restorative treatment with the easiest local analgesia, which will be an infiltration. Therefore a maxillary quadrant should be the first choice. A right-handed dentist should start with the maxillary left, and a left-handed dentist with the maxillary right. The sequence of quadrants for a right-handed dentist is then:

- first: maxillary left;
- second: maxillary right;
- third: mandibular left;
- fourth: mandibular right.

If primary incisors are involved then:

- fifth: maxillary incisors.

This approach would of course start with the right side of the mouth for a left-handed dentist because of the ease of giving an infiltration local analgesic on the opposite side of the mouth to where the dentist is sitting.

If primary *mandibular* incisors are involved then the caries rate is probably so high that a more radical approach is needed. In such cases multiple extractions are indicated, or else the approach should be restoration of the dentition under general anaesthesia.

What must be avoided is hasty restoration of badly broken down teeth in the mandible at a first visit. It is far better to dress teeth with temporary restorations (such as an intermediate restorative material and a zinc oxide and ellgenol cement, e.g. Kalzinol) and to plan the treatment in such a way as to introduce local analgesia in a controlled and simple manner so that the child readily accepts the treatment. Obviously an infiltration in the maxilla is easier to carry out than a mandibular block. Similarly an application of topical analgesic cream is easier to introduce in the maxilla.

Medical history and treatment planning

The medical history of a child will affect the type of restorative treatments that may be carried out. Obviously a full medical history should be completed for every child before dental care commences. Two specific groups of medical problems will affect which of the techniques described in this book should or should not be carried out.

Bleeding disorders

Extraction of teeth in a child with any form of bleeding disorder is contraindicated. Accordingly, for these children pulopotomies or pulpectomies are mandatory as long as the tooth is restorable.

Every effort should therefore be made to save the tooth, even to the extent of trying the various forms of pulp treatment on several occasions.

Heart conditions and immunosuppression

While over a 90% success rate can be achieved with pulpotomies and pulpectomies, there is still some risk of break down, peri-apical infection and abscess formation. Therefore in children such as those at risk of infective endocarditis with heart disease, or immunosuppression for any reason or with shunts, pulp therapy should not be carried out and any teeth with pulp involvement should be extracted, with the appropriate precautions.

Examples

To illustrate our recommended approach to treatment planning for restoration of the primary dentition, we include in Chapter 7 three cases of children treated in the way described above.

These children required extensive restorations needing several visits. They were either initially cooperative or at least took very little time to become very cooperative.

2   Local Analgesia

Introduction

Effective pain control is a prerequisite for the successful restoration of teeth. By far the most widely used technique in dentistry is the injection of local analgesic agents to block neural transmission, commonly known as 'local anaesthesia', but perhaps more correctly termed 'local analgesia'.

There are several ways of producing dental analgesia, including the use of inhalational agents, electrical nerve stimulation, general anaesthesia and hypnosis. Nevertheless, local analgesia remains the most widely used technique, being easy to administer, reliable, relatively risk-free and reasonably well tolerated by the majority of patients.

The necessity for local analgesia when restoring primary teeth has been somewhat controversial, with many dentists believing that primary teeth are 'insensitive' to pain. It is possible to successfully complete minimal restorations in some children without local anaesthesia. However, this is not true for all children—and

certainly not when more extensive restorations are required. Local analgesia is therefore to be recommended for all but the most minimal procedures such as a Type I preventive resin restoration (PRR) in a primary molar. Any dentist treating children must become skilled and confident in administering local analgesia, because without it many of the advanced techniques covered elsewhere in this book are not possible in the dental surgery.

Before the administration of local analgesia, a comprehensive medical history must be obtained so that any pre-existing medical conditions that may contraindicate the technique or the use of the drugs employed may be identified (Tables 2.1 and 2.2).

This chapter aims to illustrate some of the more useful techniques of dental local analgesia that can be successfully used in children. Consideration should also be given to avoiding overdosage of analgesic agents. Many child patients have a low body mass, and maximum dosages can easily be exceeded (Table 2.3).

Table 2.1

Conditions that may contraindicate the use of local analgesia in dentistry

Bleeding disorders	Block techniques contraindicated except with appropriate factor replacement, etc Intraligamental analgesia usually a safe alternative
Infection at injection site	Successful analgesia can often still be achieved by using a block technique
Malignant hyperpyrexia	Pre-treatment with dantrolene sodium may be necessary

Table 2.2

Conditions that may contraindicate the use of agents for local analgesia in dentistry

Lignocaine (maximum dose with vasoconstrictor 7 mg/kg)	Known hypersensitivity Acute porphyrias Heart block Epilepsy Patient taking phenytoin or propranolol
Prilocaine (maximum dose with vasoconstrictor 7 mg/kg)	Known hypersensitivity Congenital or acquired methaemoglobinaemia
Adrenaline (maximum dose 10 µg/kg, never exceeding 500 µg)	Cardiac arrhythmias Hypertension Hyperthyroidism Ischaemic heart disease Patients taking tricyclic antidepressant drugs (theoretical)
Felypressin	Pregnancy

Table 2.3

Maximum doses of commonly used local analgesic preparations in children

Age (years)	Approximate weight (kg)	Maximum dose (mg) of lignocaine or prilocaine with vasoconstrictor	Maximum dose (ml) of lignocaine 2% with 1 : 80 000 adrenaline	Maximum dose (ml) of prilocaine 3% with felypressin 0.54 µg/ml
1	10	70	3.5	2.3
5	20	140	7.0	4.6
10	30	210	10.5	7.0

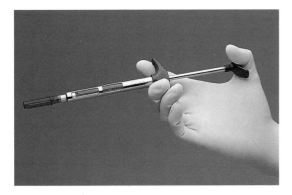

Basic principles

Armamentarium

Figure 2.1 All local analgesic injections, especially block techniques, should be performed using an aspirating syringe system.

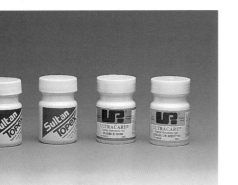

Figure 2.2 Topical analgesia. A topical analgesic should be used routinely. Benzocaine ointment 20% gives rapid and profound mucosal anaesthesia. It is available in a range of pleasant flavours, including mint, cherry, bubblegum and pina colada, and is much more readily tolerated by children than the bitter-tasting lignocaine-based products. It should be sparingly applied on a cotton roll or bud one minute before injection.

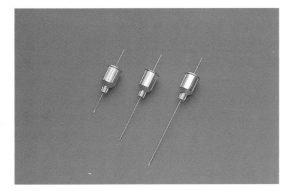

Figure 2.3 Local analgesic needle selection. A 30-gauge 2 cm needle (centre) is recommended for infiltration analgesia. A 27-gauge 3 cm needle is recommended for block techniques, where ability to aspirate is more crucial (right). For intraligamental and intrapapillary techniques a 30-gauge 1 cm needle is used (left).

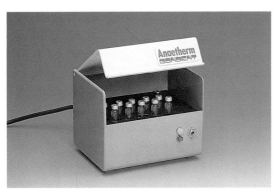

Figure 2.4 Local analgesic cartridge warmer. Warming local analgesia cartridges to body temperature helps to reduce pain during administration. Commercial warmers are available for this purpose.

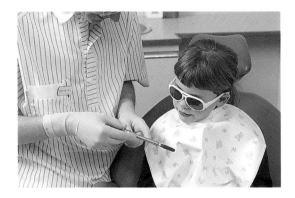

Preparation of the child for local analgesia

Figure 2.5   The child should be positioned comfortably for both child and operator. A simple explanation of the procedure should be given and, contrary to popular belief, it is often advantageous to show the child the assembled syringe, with guard in place, at this stage. This is in keeping with the 'tell–show–do' approach of behaviour management, and can be accompanied by a 'childrenese' explanation: 'Here is the jungle juice machine. In this bottle is the jungle juice and when I press this button it comes down the bottle, down a tiny tube and dribbles into your gum.' This approach will usually result in the child relaxing and accepting the administration of local without protest.

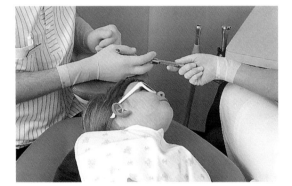

Figure 2.6   If the sight of the syringe produces anxiety in the child then this identifies a pre-existing problem, which must be appropriately managed prior to local analgesic administration. Attempts to 'hide' syringes from anxious children will frequently result in the child attempting to see what is being concealed and a heightened anxiety in both child and dentist. Any trust already established between the two may be breached.

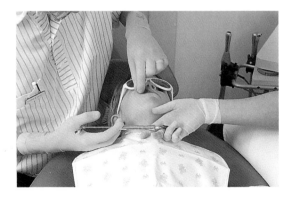

Figure 2.7   Once the explanation is complete, the needle guard can be removed, out of the child's field of vision, the soft tissues retracted and the injection carried out.

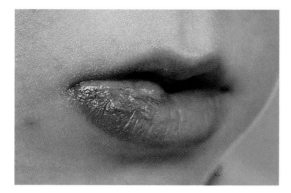

Self-inflicted soft tissue trauma

Figure 2.8 The patient must be warned not to bite, chew or suck anaesthetized lips or cheeks. The parent should also be made aware of this (since painful self-inflicted damage may result).

Infiltration analgesia

This is the most routinely used dental local analgesic technique for both restorative dentistry and minor oral surgical procedures in children. Frequently, however, additional techniques are required to secure adequate analgesia prior to treatment. Local analgesic infiltration will usually achieve pulpal analgesia in maxillary teeth, but does not reliably secure pulpal analgesia in mandibular primary molars in children of 6 years or older. (See Chapter 1.)

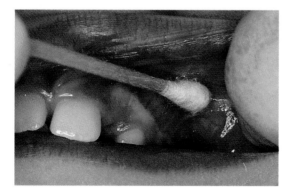

Figure 2.9 A topical analgesic agent should be applied to the mucosa for one minute prior to injection.

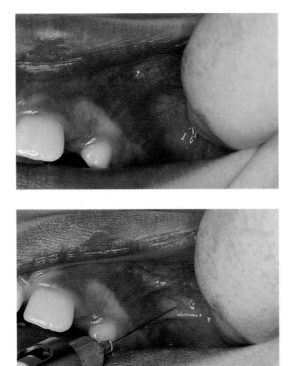

Figure 2.10 The lip/cheek should be gripped and retracted to pull the mucosa taut at the injection site.

Figure 2.11 The needle tip is advanced to the injection site and gently perforates the mucosa. This can often be achieved by 'pulling' the lip and mucosa down onto the needle. The tugging sensation produced will act as a distraction from the needle penetration.

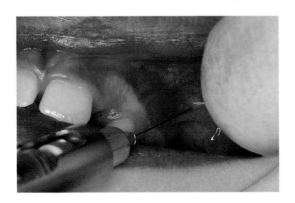

Figure 2.12 Local analgesic agent is injected *slowly*, at a rate of no more than 1 ml every 15–20 seconds. This is particularly important during the injection of the first 0.5 ml, especially in the anterior maxillary region. Aspiration should be routinely carried out at several points during the injection. Once sufficient local analgesic solution has been deposited under the mucosa, the needle should be smoothly withdrawn and the protective sheath replaced.

Maxillary molar block

This is a valuable technique, especially where infiltration is not possible because of localized infection, and produces profound analgesia of the maxillary primary/permanent molars. It results in a block of the posterior and often middle superior dental nerves as they enter the posterior maxilla in the infratemporal fossa. However, unlike the direct posterior superior nerve block technique, it does not carry the risk of damaging the vascular pterygoid plexus with subsequent haematoma formation.

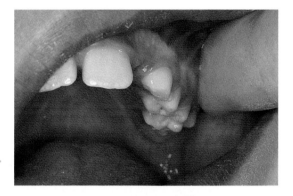

Figure 2.13 The maxillary zygomatic buttress is palpated with the index finger.

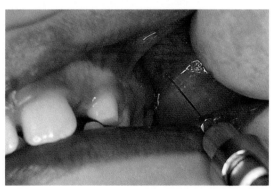

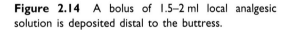

Figure 2.14 A bolus of 1.5–2 ml local analgesic solution is deposited distal to the buttress.

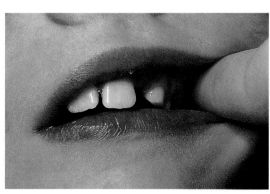

Figure 2.15 Once deposited, the analgesic solution is massaged around the distal aspect of the maxilla with the index finger. The patient should be asked to occlude at this stage. This prevents the coronoid process of the mandible blocking distal movement of the finger.

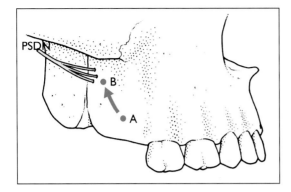

Figure 2.16 The maxillary molar block. The bolus of local analgesic solution is deposited below the mucosa distal to the zygomatic buttress (A). The analgesic solution is then massaged around the distal aspect of the maxilla into the infratemporal fossa (B) and blocking the posterior superior dental nerves (PSDN).

Palatal analgesia in children

Securing palatal analgesia is essential for extractions or rubber dam placement where the clamp will impinge on the gingivae. Traditional direct palatal injection techniques (the nasopalatine block, the greater palatine block and the palatal infiltration) are difficult to administer without significant discomfort since there is little tissue space at these sites between the mucosa and underlying periosteum. More acceptable techniques in children are the intrapapillary and indirect palatal injections.

Intrapapillary injection

This provides suitable palatal analgesia for rubber dam, matrix band or stainless steel crown placement on all maxillary primary teeth. It will also give adequate analgesia for extraction of primary incisors and canines. It will produce the same effect in the lower arch in children of 5 years of age and below where infiltration rather than block analgesia has been administered.

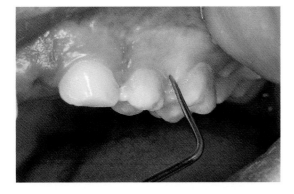

Figure 2.17 A buccal infiltration injection is administered. After approximately two minutes, analgesia of the buccal aspect of the interdental papillae mesial and distal to the tooth is tested with a probe.

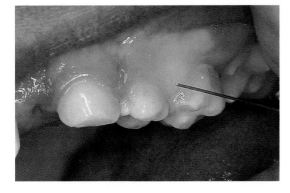

Figure 2.18 The interdental papilla is penetrated using a 30-gauge needle to a depth of 1–2 mm. The syringe barrel is held parallel to the occlusal plane and perpendicular to the line of the arch. Local analgesic solution is injected slowly, and the needle is gently advanced to a depth of a few millimetres.

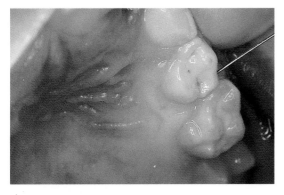

Figure 2.19 Injection should continue until blanching of the palate is observed extending more than halfway along the palatal gingival margin. This usually takes 20–30 seconds.

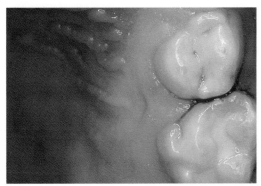

Figure 2.20 The same procedure is repeated on the other side of the tooth, with injection continuing until the blanching extends to and joins with that produced by the previous injection. Analgesia of the complete gingival cuff has now been achieved.

Indirect palatal injection

In young children more profound palatal analgesia, suitable for the extraction of maxillary molars, may be achieved by an indirect palatal technique. This is similar to the intrapapillary technique, but the needle is angled slightly upwards and, while it is injected, advanced through the interdental papilla, below the contact and beneath the palatal mucosa. A bolus of analgesic solution can be deposited palatally.

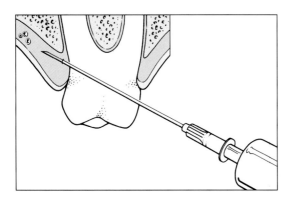

Figure 2.21   Indirect palatal injection.

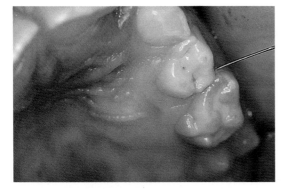

Figure 2.22   Blanching of the palatal mucosa, demonstrating final site of local analgesic solution deposition.

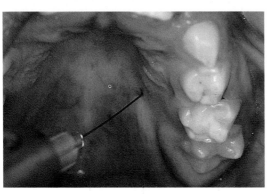

Figure 2.23   Analgesia can be further reinforced painlessly by direct palatal infiltration once indirect analgesia has been achieved.

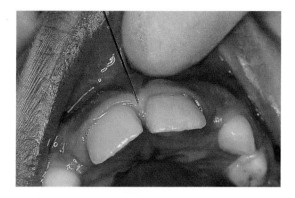

Figure 2.24 The indirect approach is particularly useful prior to the administration of a nasopalatine block.

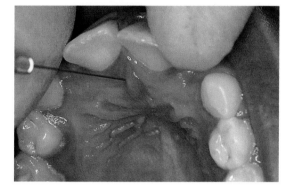

Figure 2.25 The nasopalatine block is painlessly administered using the standard technique, analgesia of the nasopalatine papilla having been previously secured by an indirect palatal approach.

Inferior dental block

The inferior dental block is recommended for all procedures in mandibular primary molars requiring pulpal analgesia in children of 6 years or older. A 27-gauge needle is recommended for more reliable aspiration.

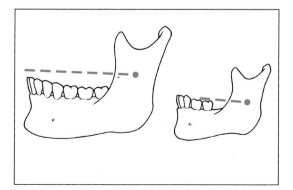

Figure 2.26 The child's mandibular foramen lies relatively lower and deeper along the internal surface of the ascending ramus when compared with that in an adult.

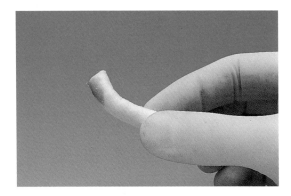

Figure 2.27 Topical analgesia is most reliably achieved by placing topical gel on the outer aspect of a bent cotton roll.

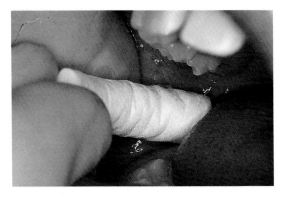

Figure 2.28 The gel is placed in contact with the tissues overlying the injection site.

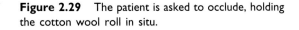

Figure 2.29 The patient is asked to occlude, holding the cotton wool roll in situ.

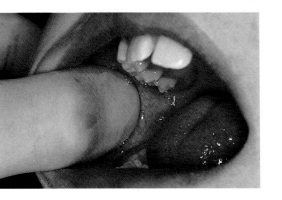

Figure 2.30 The patient is instructed to open the mouth as wide as possible. The thumb palpates the external oblique ridge and tautens the mucosa between the pterygomandibular raphe and the external oblique ridge.

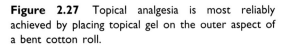

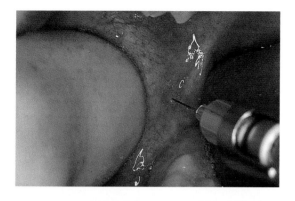

Figure 2.31 The needle is inserted from the opposite side of the mouth, the barrel lying over the first primary molar. The needle enters the tissues at a point midway between the external oblique ridge and the pterygomandibular raphe at the level of the occlusal plane. Once the mucosa has been penetrated a small amount of analgesic solution is immediately deposited; the needle is then gently advanced, with slow injection and aspiration until the resistance of the bone of the internal surface of the ramus is felt. The periosteum at this site is sensitive, and so great care should be exercised. The needle is withdrawn 1 mm and the remainder of the solution slowly deposited.

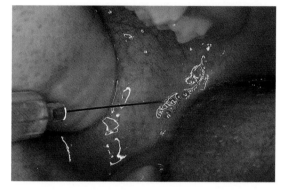

Figure 2.32 In young children a two-stage technique may be preferred for inferior dental block administration. This involves first giving a small submucosal infiltration at the injection site.

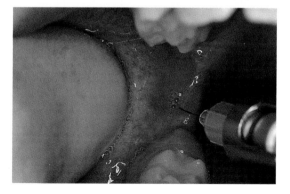

Figure 2.33 After 1–2 minutes, an inferior dental block can be administered, injecting through the already anaesthetized tissues.

Intraligamental techniques

The intraligamental technique is an effective method of achieving pulpal analgesia in both primary and permanent teeth, especially where routine infiltration or block techniques have failed. In spite of its name, the local analgesic solution is introduced via the periodontium, travelling down the periodontal space. The majority of solution deposited escapes through the lamina dura into cancellous bone. It is therefore in some ways similar to an intraosseous injection.

Some writers have voiced concern about potential damage to developing permanent teeth due to the high pressures produced within the periodontium when this technique is used on primary teeth, especially molars. Although this is a theoretical possibility, at the time of writing the authors are unaware of any substantiated cases of such damage in the literature.

Recent evidence shows that the intraligamental injection produces a significant transient bacteraemia on virtually every occasion it is administered. Hence it is contraindicated in patients at risk from such bacteraemias. In addition, solutions containing adrenaline should be avoided in patients with a history of hypertension or cardiac arrhythmias, since the technique is frequently accompanied by a rapid rise in plasma adrenaline levels.

The technique is contraindicated where significant periodontal disease or acute periodontal inflammation is present. Any gross plaque should be cleared from the site prior to injection.

Several commercial syringes are available for the intraligamental injection technique. Although it is possible to administer an intraligamental injection with a standard syringe, the high pressures produced in the cartridge may cause it to fracture, with potentially serious consequences. Purpose-designed syringe systems have shielded barrels to support the cartridge and prevent loss of glass fragments, should it fracture.

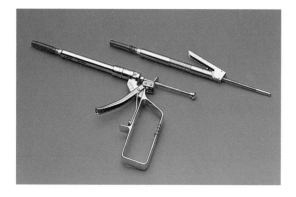

Figure 2.34 The Peripress (left) and Paraject intraligamental syringes. The authors prefer the latter for use in children, since it is smaller and less threatening in appearance. Similar pen-like designs are available from other manufacturers.

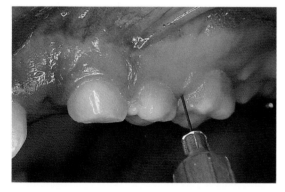

Figure 2.35 A 30-gauge 1 cm needle is used for intraligamental injections. It is introduced into the interproximal periodontal sulcus at approximately 50–60° to the occlusal plane, and is gently advanced into the periodontal space for about 5–6 mm or until firm bony resistance is felt.

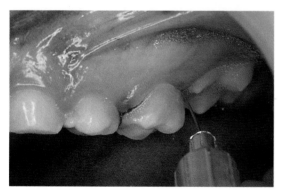

Figure 2.36 Injection is commenced, using firm, steady pressure and noting the presence of significant resistance or 'back-pressure'. If significant back-pressure is not encountered, the needle should be withdrawn and reinserted at a slightly different point, and the injection tried again. About 0.4–0.6 ml should be deposited both mesially and distally to the tooth. Analgesia, if successful, is almost immediate.

3   Rubber Dam

Unlike many of the techniques used in modern restorative dentistry, rubber dam is not a recent innovation. Its use was described by Barnum as early as 1865 in the *British Journal of Dental Science*.

Rubber dam is rarely used in routine dentistry in the UK. A recent survey revealed that only 1.4% of UK dentists use it on a routine basis. More surprisingly, only 11% used it most or all of the time for endodontics, even though it is widely recommended to protect patients from accidental inhalation or ingestion of small instruments.

Rubber dam has many advantages, in addition to airway protection (Table 3.1). Effective isolation is essential for many restorative procedures. Rubber dam provides a dry, contamination-free field and retracts and protects the soft tissues against accidental damage. These conditions are often difficult to achieve in the mouths of young children by alternative methods. Rubber dam is well tolerated by both children and adults, with the majority of patients preferring to have it used for restorative procedures once they have experienced the improvement in intra-operative comfort. If used properly, rubber dam is both easy and quick to use, saving far more time during almost all operative procedures than it actually takes to apply.

It has recently been demonstrated that rubber dam is also an excellent aid to cross-infection control. The contamination of the area immediately surrounding the patient's head by oral microorganisms can be reduced by 95–99% during air rotor and triple syringe use with a rubber dam in situ when compared with the same procedures without dam. The aim of this chapter is to demonstrate simple and versatile techniques for the application of rubber dam in children. Common problems and their solutions will also be presented.

Table 3.1

Advantages of rubber dam

Moisture-free operating field

Isolation from salivary contamination

Improved access

Protection and retraction of soft tissues

Improved patient comfort

Minimized procedural time

Minimized mouthbreathing (especially useful when inhalation sedation is being administered)

Reduced risk of inhalation or ingestion of small instruments or debris

Cross-infection control is achieved by minimization of aerosol spread of microorganisms

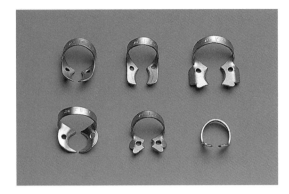

Armamentarium

Figure 3.1 Clamps. A wide range of clamps is available from several manufacturers. The majority of situations encountered in children can be adequately catered for by a small selection of clamp patterns. The clamps detailed and illustrated are from the Ash range (Ash Instruments, Dentsply, Addlestone, Surrey, UK), but similar and equally suitable patterns are available from other manufacturers, such as Hygenic and Hu Freidy. DW (top left): this is ideal for first and second primary molars, and is suitable for some central incisors. BW (top centre): this is suitable for larger second primary molars and first permanent molars. K (top right): this is a winged clamp for larger, fully erupted first permanent molars, especially lower first molars when several teeth are to be isolated utilizing the trough technique. FW (bottom left): this is a retentive clamp that is especially useful for partially erupted first permanent molars. L (bottom centre): this is suitable for small first primary molars. EW (bottom right): this is suitable for small premolars and primary canines and incisors.

Figure 3.2 Rubber dam is available in a variety of colours and thicknesses (or grades). Some of the coloured dams are also flavoured to mask the latex taste, making them particularly suitable for children. Medium grade (which confusingly is the thinnest of the three grades generally available) is the most suitable thickness for the techniques described below.

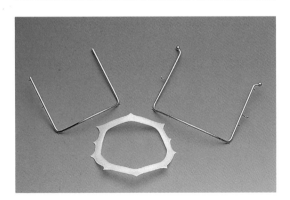

Figure 3.3 Several rubber dam frames are available. The Ash pattern (right), based on the original Young's pattern, is the most suitable for children. The modified Young's pattern (left) and the Svenska N-Ø frame (bottom) are also shown.

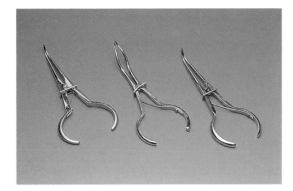

Figure 3.4   A variety of clamp placement forceps are available. Three popular patterns are shown   here: Stokes (left), Brewer (middle) and Ash (right). The Ash pattern (Ash Instruments, Dentsply, Addlestone, Surrey, UK) is recommended for children, since it will securely lock open when holding small clamps, and the straight arms provide the easiest access to small mouths.

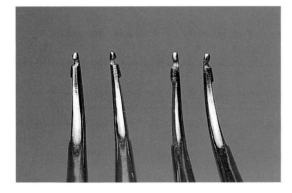

Figure 3.5   The beaks of some patterns of forceps are manufactured with grooves in their outer surfaces to ensure positive location of the clamp during expansion and placement. Unfortunately, the shape of the beak below this groove can impede removal of the forceps once the clamp has been placed (left). This problem can be avoided by simple modification of the beak tips by grinding with an abrasive stone (right).

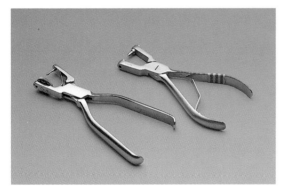

Figure 3.6   The traditional punch for making holes in rubber dam is the Ainsworth pattern (left). This incorporates a rotating wheel, which allows the selection of different hole sizes. Unfortunately, because of its complexity, this punch often deteriorates rapidly with repeated sterilization. This, coupled with the fact that one size of hole is usually adequate for most situations, has led the authors to adopt the much simpler Ash pattern punch (right) for routine use. This has the added advantage that the jaws can be removed and replaced at minimal cost if they become damaged.

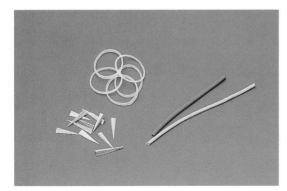

Figure 3.7   Additional retention can be obtained by a number of devices, including wooden wedges, orthodontic elastics and commercially available latex cord (Wedjets: Hygenic Corporation, Ohio, USA).

Contraindications/cautions regarding the use of rubber dam

There are few situations when rubber dam should not be used. The only absolute contraindication is known allergy to latex. Rarely, application of rubber dam will produce an allergic reaction in an individual previously not known to be sensitized to latex. These reactions may vary in severity from mild contact dermatitis to severe hypersensitivity. However, even this problem can be overcome if necessary by using food-quality polythene sheeting. Caution should also be exercised in patients at risk from transient bacteraemia, such as those with congenital heart defects or immunosuppression. If gingival trauma is unavoidable, suitable antibiotic prophylaxis should be administered. Severe gingival disease may also contraindicate dam placement.

Preparation of the child patient for rubber dam

Rubber dam should be introduced to the child in just the same way as any other routine part of the dental procedure. The dam can be presented as a 'raincoat' that keeps the tooth dry and is held on by a 'button' (clamp) and kept straight by a 'coat hanger' (frame). Sun glasses and a suitable bib should be placed on the child to protect the eyes and clothing.

Local analgesia should be administered in any situation where a clamp may impinge on the gingivae. This is particularly important when clamping primary molars since the maximum bulbosity of the crown lies just above the gingival margin and some pressure on the gingivae is virtually unavoidable. Pain caused by clamp pressure on unanaesthetized gingivae is one of the commonest reasons for children disliking dam. Analgesia of the complete pericoronal gingival cuff must be secured. Infiltration plus intra-papillary injections or, in the lower arch, an inferior dental block will achieve this effectively (Chapter 2).

A mouth prop may be used to help the child maintain an open mouth. This can be introduced as a 'cushion to rest your teeth on'. Some patients find this beneficial, whereas others prefer treatment without it.

Single molar isolation

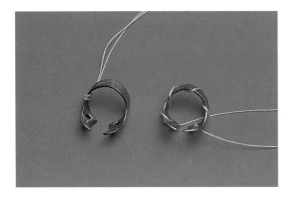

Figure 3.8 A suitable clamp is selected (Figure 3.1). Floss is secured around the clamp to assist its retrieval should it come loose in the mouth. This can be achieved either by looping round the bow or by passing the floss through the forceps holes and spiralling around the bow. The latter technique was devised to avoid loss of the clamp should it break in two in the mouth. However, this is time-consuming, and floss trails from both sides of the clamp, often causing a nuisance during restorative care. The floss can also inadvertently be cut by pressure from the forcep beaks during placement, rendering it useless. The introduction of anodized clamps has reduced the risk of corrosion fracture, and hence such elaborate precautions may be unnecessary, attachment of floss to the bow being adequate.

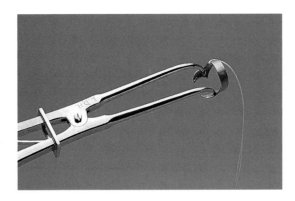

Figure 3.9 The clamp is placed on the forceps, expanded and the forceps locked.

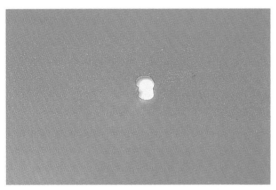

Figure 3.10 A sheet of medium-grade rubber dam is selected and a double overlapping hole is punched in it. In the primary dentition the hole should be near the middle of the dam, whichever tooth is to be clamped. When clamping first and second permanent molars in older children, the hole should be punched nearer the top of the dam for upper teeth and nearer the bottom for lower teeth.

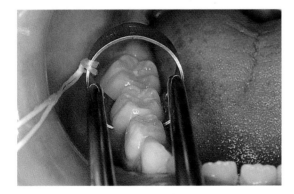

Figure 3.11 The clamp is placed onto the tooth to be isolated, and carefully positioned at the gingival margin. The locking sleeve of the clamp forceps is released, and the clamp is allowed to grip the tooth.

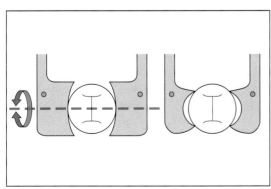

Figure 3.12 Before removing the forceps, the stability of the clamp is checked, ensuring that good four-point contact with the tooth is achieved (right). If only two-point contact is obtained, the clamp will rock and be unstable (left).

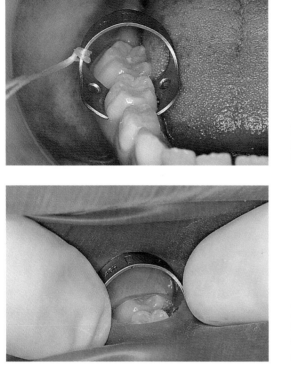

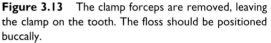

Figure 3.13   The clamp forceps are removed, leaving the clamp on the tooth. The floss should be positioned buccally.

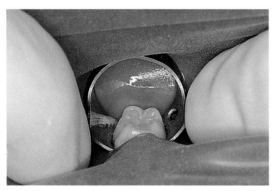

Figure 3.14   The rubber dam sheet is carried into the mouth, with both index fingers being used to stretch the hole and position it over the bow of the clamp.

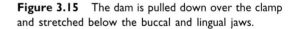

Figure 3.15   The dam is pulled down over the clamp and stretched below the buccal and lingual jaws.

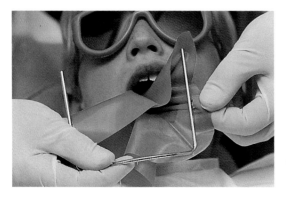

Figure 3.16   The frame is then placed, first stretching the lower dam onto the bottom corners then hooking it onto the upper prongs. The aim is to have the isolated tooth positioned equidistant between the two sides of the frame, with the top ends of the frame just below the level of the nostrils.

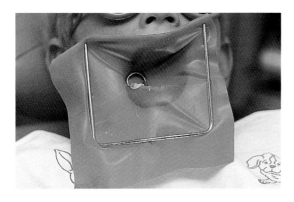

Figure 3.17 The dam is finally stretched over the remaining prongs on the frame.

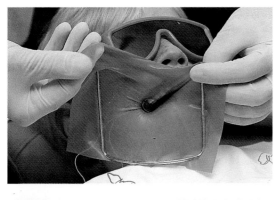

Figure 3.18 If there is excess dam at the top edge, as often occurs when upper teeth are isolated, this can be easily reflected and tucked under the top edge of the frame.

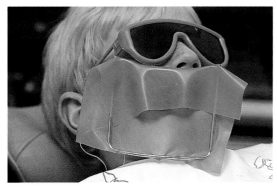

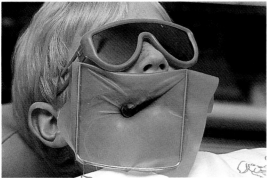

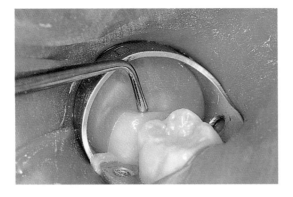

Figure 3.19 If the dam has caught on the cusp on an adjacent tooth, it should be teased into place with a round-ended burnisher, taking care not to tear the dam.

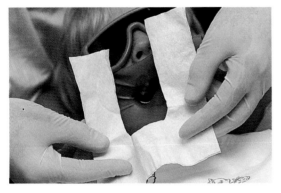

Figure 3.20 Optionally, a U-shaped piece of absorbent tissue can be tucked under the dam from below. This helps to absorb moisture and improves patient comfort.

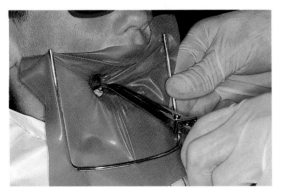

Figure 3.21 Once restorative work is complete, the forceps are re-engaged in the clamp holes, and the clamp, dam and frame are removed in one procedure.

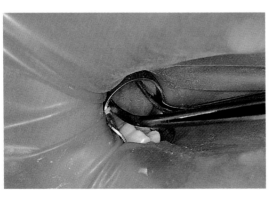

Figure 3.22 Alternatively, the forceps beaks may be inserted inverted into the bow of the clamp and expanded to remove the clamp. Most dam clamp forceps have flattened necks on the beaks to facilitate this.

Quadrant isolation: the trough technique

Frequently, more than one tooth in a quadrant requires restoration, or access to interproximal caries is necessary. The trough technique provides an excellent method of achieving this in children. Although it does not give the absolute isolation that can be achieved with a more classical individual hole technique, it is quick, easy and reliable, making it ideal for routine use.

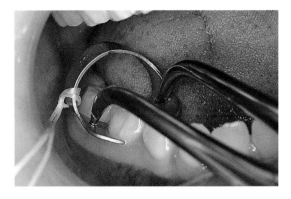

Figure 3.23 The clamp is placed on the most distal tooth to be isolated, as in the single-tooth technique. Here the second primary molar is clamped, but if extensive treatment is planned on this tooth then the first permanent molar should be clamped if erupted.

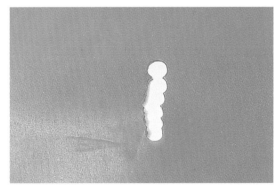

Figure 3.24 A row of overlapping holes is punched in the middle of the dam, creating a trough about 10–15 mm long.

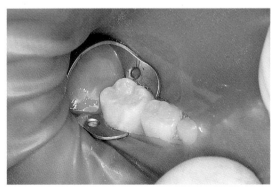

Figure 3.25 The trough is stretched over the clamp as before and the frame placed.

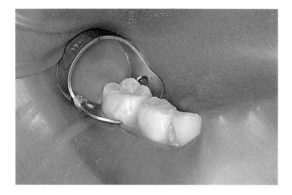

Figure 3.26   The dam is now stretched forward and hooked over the primary canine. The dam will usually retain itself in this position, isolating the molars and canine.

Additional retention

If necessary, additional retention can be achieved anteriorly by several methods.

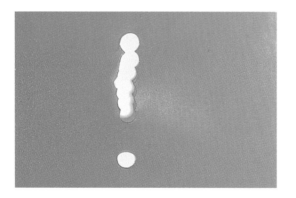

Figure 3.27   An additional hole can be punched about 5 mm beyond the anterior end of the trough.

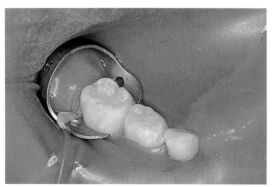

Figure 3.28   This hole can be stretched over the primary canine, with the dam passing between the latter and the first molar; this helps to retain the dam.

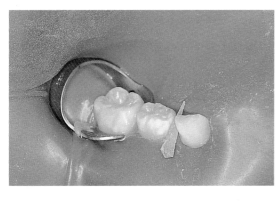

Figure 3.29 Wooden wedges may be inserted inter-proximally to retain the dam.

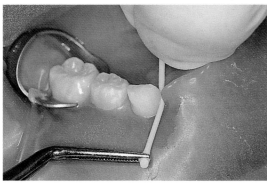

Figure 3.30 Commercially available latex cord (Wedjets: Hygenic Corporation, Ohio, USA) can be stretched and passed through the contact area.

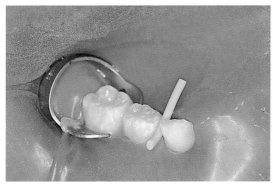

Figure 3.31 Once released, the strips expand and lock the dam into position.

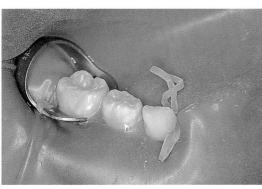

Figure 3.32 Orthodontic elastic bands can be used in a similar fashion.

Upper incisor teeth

There are several methods of isolating upper incisor teeth in the primary and early mixed dentition.

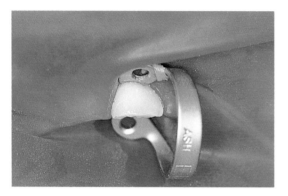

Figure 3.33 Individual primary incisor teeth can be clamped with an EW clamp.

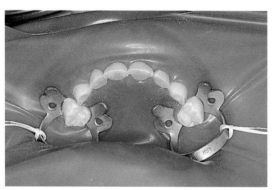

Figure 3.34 All six upper anterior teeth can be isolated using two clamps applied to the first primary molars. In this situation the dam is applied first and then the clamps placed to stabilize it.

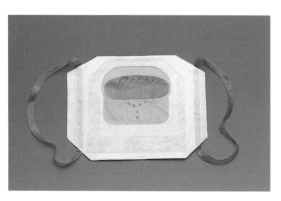

Figure 3.35 A prefabricated semi-rigid dam and tissue unit (Dry Dam: Svenska AB, Sweden) provides a useful alternative for upper anterior teeth. This preformed dam includes retention elastics that hook round the patient's ears to hold the sheet in place.

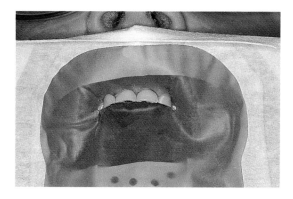

Figure 3.36 Although additional stabilization with fingers or wedges is sometimes necessary, clamping is not usually required.

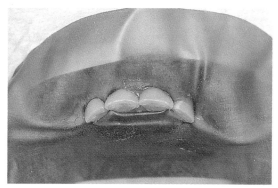

Figure 3.37 Where interproximal access is required, this may be facilitated by cutting the interproximal dam to join two holes and create a 'trough'.

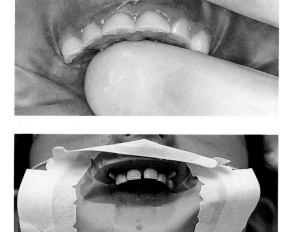

Figure 3.38 In small children a simple slot rather than individual holes will often provide a quick and practical way of isolating several incisors.

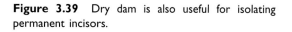

Figure 3.39 Dry dam is also useful for isolating permanent incisors.

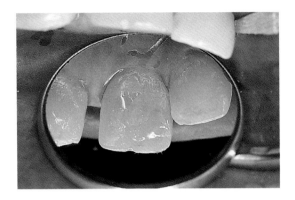

Figure 3.40 The excellent access to the palatal aspect of the incisor—necessary, for example, if endodontics is planned—is clearly demonstrated.

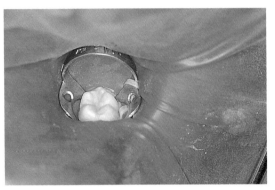

Figure 3.41 Partially erupted first permanent molars are usually best clamped using the FW clamp.

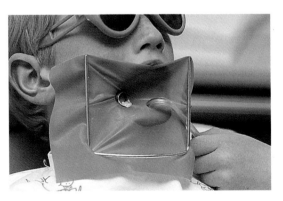

Figure 3.42 If suction beneath the dam is required, this can be best achieved by passing a flexible aspirator tip through an additional hole in the rubber dam.

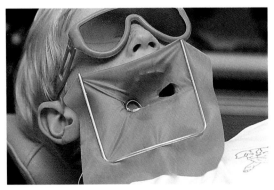

Figure 3.43 Occasionally, patients will complain that they cannot breathe with the dam in place. This may be a particular problem for asthmatics. It can be solved by simply cutting a hole in the dam, away from the operating site. If the hole is sited correctly, isolation and airway protection should not be significantly compromised.

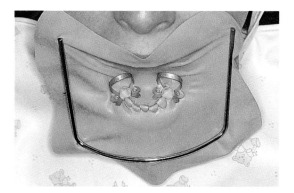

Figure 3.44 Lower incisors are difficult to isolate, in both primary and permanent dentitions. The use of individual holes, with placement of the dam first and clamps second, usually provides the most satisfactory result.

4 Pulp Therapy for Primary Teeth

In spite of the decline in the prevalence of dental caries in children in the western world, there is still a large population where caries is still rampant (Figure 4.1). It is therefore important for all dental practitioners to be familiar with the techniques for maintaining and restoring the primary teeth. Preservation of primary teeth in the arch is important both for the management of the developing dentition and in nurturing a positive attitude in children towards dental health. Extraction of primary teeth just because they are 'baby teeth' or 'first teeth', without any thought to the long-term development of the dentition and the child, is no longer defensible. In addition to preserving the arch form, the use of pulp therapy to conserve carious primary teeth may:

- allow preservation of a pulpally involved primary molar when the permanent successor is missing;
- prevent possible aberrant habits, such as tongue habits;
- maintain masticatory function;
- preserve aesthetics.

Most importantly, by conserving the primary teeth, the dentist sends a message to both the parent and the child that teeth are important and should be retained. To extract teeth without making an effort to preserve them suggests that they are unimportant, with a possible bearing on the future dental attitudes of both parent and child.

It is therefore up to the dental practitioner to make all efforts to conserve primary teeth. Techniques are available to preserve teeth even with pulpal involvement and infection that has led to abscesses. Most primary molars can be conserved provided that there remains sufficient crown tissue to retain the final restoration.

The purpose of this chapter is to help in the understanding of the indications of pulp therapy in primary teeth and to present a clear, step-by-step method of carrying out the procedures involved in pulp treatment.

A. THE PULPOTOMY TECHNIQUE

A pulpotomy is the procedure of removing the coronal part of the pulp tissue, inflamed or infected, as a result of deep caries, and the maintenance of vital radicular pulp tissue. A

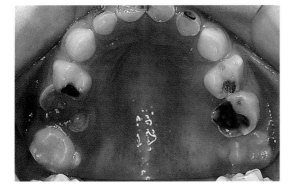

Figure 4.1 Intra-oral photograph showing multiple carious lesions in the primary teeth. This is a common feature in many children presenting for treatment.

medicament is applied to the remaining root tissue with the aim of 'fixing' it. Currently the most widely accepted material, supported by a large number of research studies, is a 1/5 dilution of the original Buckley's formocresol, the constituents of which are shown in Table 4.1.

Table 4.1
Constituents of the original Buckley's formocresol

Tricresol	35%
Formaldehyde	19%
Glycerol	15%
Water	31%

Research has shown that the full-strength solution shown in table 4.1 is unnecessary, and a 1/5 dilution is as successful. The dilute solution is constituted as shown in Table 4.2. This is enough for a large number of pulpotomies.

Table 4.2
Method of preparing a 1/5 dilution of formocresol

Buckley's formocresol	30 ml
Glycerol	90 ml
Water	30 ml

Diagnosis

Many clinicians seem to have difficulty in deciding whether a pulpotomy should be carried out on a primary tooth with deep caries. It is very tempting, especially with the widespread use of glass ionomer cements, to remove caries with a slow-speed handpiece and a round bur and place one of these cements in the cavity. The fluoride-releasing properties of glass ionomers are thought to have a protective effect, even if some caries is left

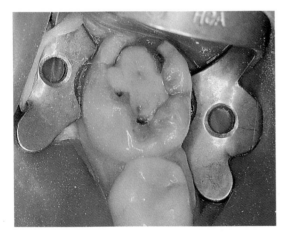

Figure 4.2 A failed glass ionomer restoration performed without complete removal of caries. The leaching of fluoride into the cavity does not stop the progression of caries.

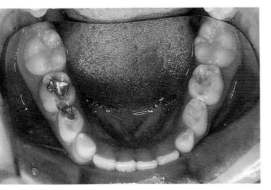

Figure 4.3 Example of failed amalgam restorations performed without administration of local analgesia.

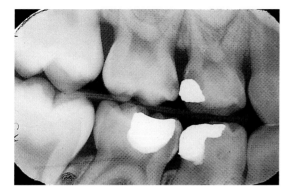

Figure 4.4 Radiograph of patient in Figure 4.3 showing residual caries.

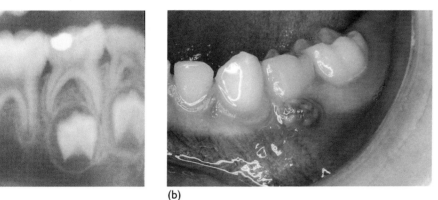

(a)   (b)

Figure 4.5 (a) Radiograph showing loss of bone in the bifurcation area under 85 inadequately restored with a glass ionomer cement. (b) Abscess in relation to 74 that had a glass ionomer filling placed without local analgesia and incomplete removal of caries.

in the tooth. This is a misconception, and experience has shown that it is a recipe for disaster and that most of these restorations will fail (Figure 4.2), with the same being true for amalgam restorations placed without complete removal of caries (Figures 4.3 and 4.4). A large proportion of teeth restored in such a manner will develop abscesses (Figure 4.5). The reason for this is that caries in primary teeth compromises the pulp very early on, with pulp inflammation setting in even before the pulp is exposed. The classical studies by Hobson (1970) showed that in over 50% of primary molars where loss of the marginal ridge had occurred pulp inflammation was irreversible. Most primary teeth where the marginal ridge is involved in the carious process will therefore require a pulpotomy. Because of this early inflammation of the coronal pulp in primary teeth, *direct pulp capping is contraindicated*. This point is illustrated in Figures 4.6–4.9.

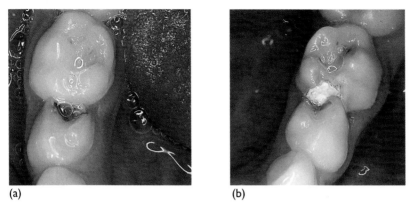

(a)   (b)

Figure 4.6   (a, b) Photographs showing the involvement of the marginal ridge of primary molars. The coronal pulp is probably inflamed in these teeth, and a pulpotomy is indicated.

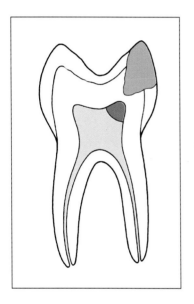

Figure 4.7   Illustration showing early involvement of the pulp in primary molars under a carious lesion. The coronal pulp tissue is usually inflamed even before the pulp is exposed.

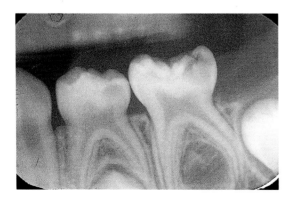

Figure 4.8   Radiograph showing large distal lesions in both 74 and 75. Even though there is no radiographic pulp exposure, the coronal pulp tissue is probably inflamed, and these teeth require a pulpotomy.

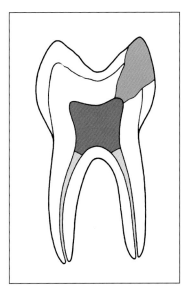

Figure 4.9 By the time the caries exposes the pulp, the inflammation is irreversible. Direct pulp capping with calcium hydroxide will only perpetuate the inflammation, and is contraindicated. A pulpotomy is therefore indicated, with the aim being removal of the affected coronal pulp and preservation of vital radicular pulp tissue.

Indications for pulpotomy

- Large carious lesion with substantial loss (one-third or more) of the marginal ridge in an otherwise restorable tooth.
- Tooth free of radicular pulpitis. This is established by the following:
  (a) History—no history of spontaneous or persistent pain. This would imply irreversible pulpitis extending to the radicular tissue.
  (b) Haemorrhage from amputation site—after removal of coronal pulp, the haemorrhage from the root canal tissue should be pale red and easy to control. Extensive and persistent bleeding implies inflammation of the radicular tissue.
- At least two-thirds of the root length of the primary tooth still present.
- Absence of an abscess or fistula.
- No inter-radicular bone loss. Any loss would suggest a more extensive involvement, indicating the need for a pulpectomy (Section B of this chapter).
- No evidence of internal resorption in either the pulp chamber or the root canal.
- Instances where extraction of the primary tooth is contraindicated, such as in some blood dyscrasias (e.g. haemophilia).

Contraindications for pulpotomy

- An unrestorable tooth.
- Bi- or trifurcation involvement or the presence of an abscess.
- Less than two-thirds of the root remaining.
- Permanent successor close to eruption.

Medical contraindications

- *Heart disease*: a pulpotomy should not be performed in a child with a heart defect, or if there is any history of heart disease, heart surgery, rheumatic fever etc. This is because these children are at risk of developing bacterial endocarditis from any invasive procedures.
- *Immuno-compromised children*, such as those with malignant disease (e.g. leukaemia) who are neutropenic for considerable periods during the treatment of the condition. Even a low-grade infection such as that from an unsuccessful pulpotomy can make such children seriously ill, and therefore should not be undertaken.

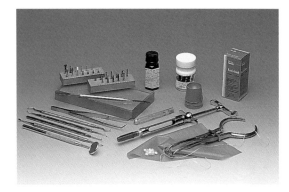

Armamentarium for the pulpotomy technique

Figure 4.10 The armamentarium comprises the following: topical and local analgesics; burs No 330 FG high speed and No 8 RA slow speed; dappens pot; syringe; zinc oxide eugenol (Kalzinol); rubber dam kit; mouth mirror, probe and tweezers; cotton pellets (small); large and small excavators; mixing spatula; flat plastic instrument; formocresol, 1/5 dilution.

The step-by-step pulpotomy technique

A thorough pre-operative assessment should be carried out by taking a good history, clinical examination and radiographs.

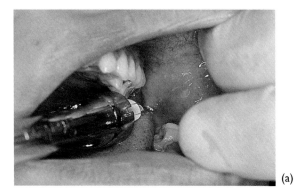

(a)

Step 1: Administer local analgesia with the use of a topical analgesic

Figure 4.11 It is essential to achieve profound analgesia. This would usually mean an inferior dental nerve block for lower teeth and an infiltration for the upper teeth (Chapter 2). For lower primary molars, in addition to a nerve block (a), a buccal infiltration (b) should always be given to anaesthetize the long buccal nerve for the placement of the rubber dam clamp.

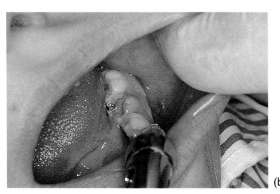

(b)

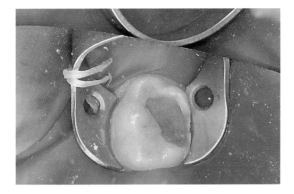

Step 2: Isolate tooth with rubber dam

Figure 4.12 This shows 75 isolated with a rubber dam. This is important to prevent any further contamination of the pulp, to aid patient comfort and to prevent leakage of formocresol onto the soft tissues.

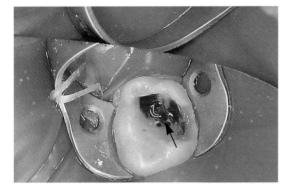

Step 3: Remove caries and determine site of pulp exposure

Figure 4.13 It is important to remove all visible caries before the pulp chamber is entered, otherwise bleeding from the pulp will make visualization of caries difficult. It is also necessary to determine the exposure site (arrow), since it is easier to gain access to the pulp chamber through the exposure.

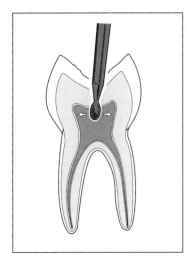

(a)

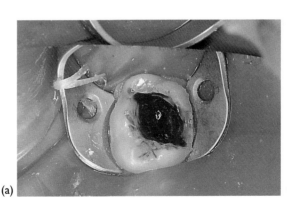

(b)

Step 4: Remove roof of pulp chamber

Figure 4.14 The bur is placed in the exposure, and the site is widened until the whole of the roof of the chamber is removed. If there is no apparent exposure, the cavity is made deeper until a 'dip' is felt, when the bur passes through the roof into the void of the pulp chamber. Once the pulp chamber has been entered, the bur is not taken any deeper but is moved sideways to remove the roof of the chamber (a). Haemorrhage from the pulp will be evident at this stage (b).

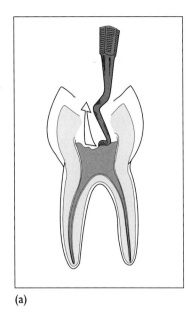

(a)

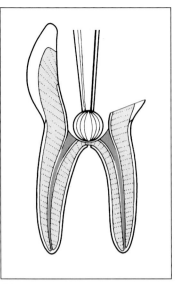

(b)

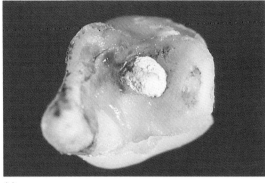

(c)

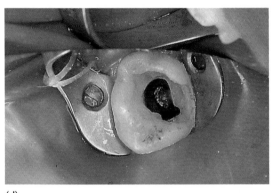

(d)

Step 5: Remove coronal pulp with a large excavator or a large round bur

Figure 4.15 A large excavator is preferred to remove the coronal pulp tissue (a). When a round bur is used, care must be taken that it is only moved lightly along the floor of the pulp chamber. Any excessive pressure can result in perforation of the floor and failure of the pulpotomy (b, c). After removal of the inflamed coronal tissue, the haemorrhage into the cavity should be reduced (d).

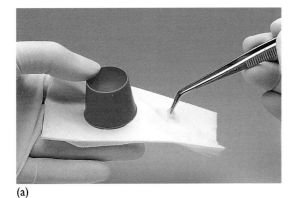

(a)

Step 6: Apply formocresol on a pledget of cotton wool for four minutes

Figure 4.16 A small pledget of cotton wool is dipped in formocresol and squeezed in a piece of gauze to remove excess (a) before it is placed in the pulp chamber for four minutes (b).

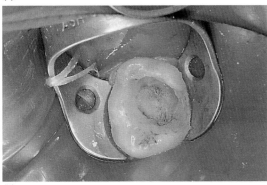

(b)

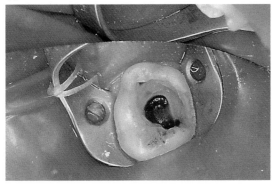

Step 7: Remove formocresol pledget after four minutes and check that the haemorrhage has stopped

Figure 4.17 Continued bleeding from the root canal tissue signifies inflammation of the radicular tissue. If this occurs the pulp should be extirpated and a pulpectomy performed as described in Section B of this chapter.

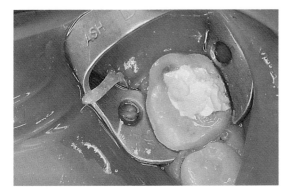

Step 8: Fill pulp chamber with cement

Figure 4.18 When the haemorrhage has been arrested, the pulp chamber is filled with one of the proprietary brands of zinc oxide eugenol, such as Kalzinol.

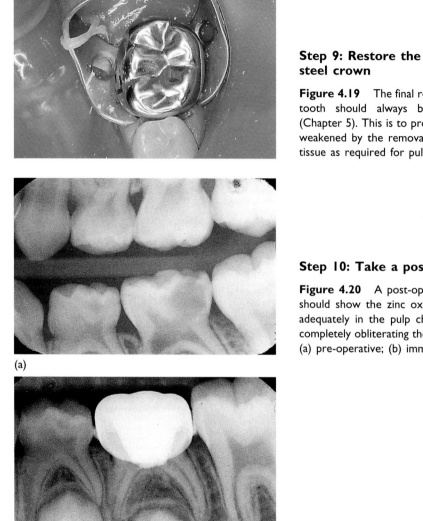

(a)

(b)

Step 9: Restore the tooth with a stainless steel crown

Figure 4.19 The final restoration of any pulp-treated tooth should always be a stainless steel crown (Chapter 5). This is to provide protection to the tooth weakened by the removal of a large amount of tooth tissue as required for pulp therapy.

Step 10: Take a postoperative radiograph

Figure 4.20 A post-operative peri-apical radiograph should show the zinc oxide eugenol filling condensed adequately in the pulp chamber of 75 and preferably completely obliterating the openings of the root canals: (a) pre-operative; (b) immediately post-operative.

Follow-up

Teeth that have undergone pulpotomy should be regularly reviewed both clinically and radiographically at follow-up visits, preferably 6-monthly. Periapical radiographs or good bitewings that allow visualization of the furcation area should be taken.

Appearance of rarefaction of the bone in the furcation area or a worsening of the bone condition in the furcation usually signifies failure of the procedure. A decision is then made to either extract the tooth, carry out a pulpectomy or observe for a few months, on the basis of other clinical considerations such as behaviour and space requirements.

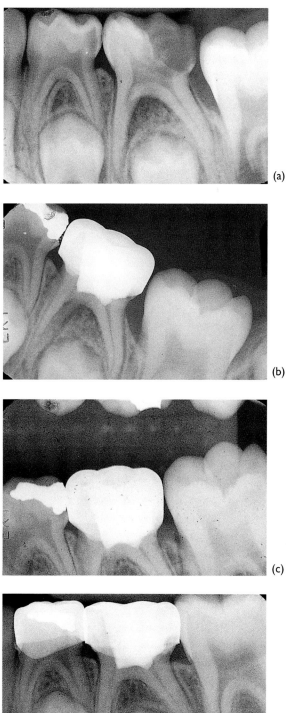

(a)

(b)

(c)

(d)

Figure 4.21 A series of follow-up radiographs after a pulpotomy was carried out on 75: (a) pre-operative; (b) immediately post-operative; (c) three months; (d) 12 months. There has been no deterioration of the bone in the bifurcation region, an indication of success.

Mechanism of action of formocresol

Since the 1950s, much work has been done to evaluate the effect of formocresol on pulp tissue, including histological, biochemical and histochemical enzymatic studies. Essentially, formocresol acts through the aldehyde group of formaldehyde, forming bonds with the side-groups of the amino acids of both the bacterial proteins and those of the remaining pulp tissue. It is therefore both a bactericidal and devitalizing agent. It kills off and converts bacteria and pulp tissue into inert compounds.

It has also been shown that formocresol inactivates the oxidative enzymes in the pulp tissue adjacent to the amputation site. It may also have some effect on hyaluronidase action. Therefore the protein-binding properties and the inhibition of the enzymes that can break the pulp tissue down together result in 'fixation' of the pulp tissue by formocresol and render it inert and resistant to enzymatic breakdown.

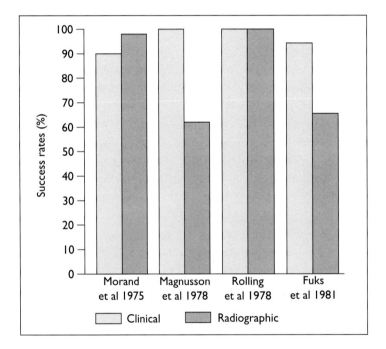

Reported success rate of formocresol pulpotomy

Figure 4.22 Histogram showing the reported clinical and radiographic success rates of formocresol pulpotomies followed up between three and five years.

Alternatives to formocresol

There has recently been concern about the possible toxicity of formocresol, both locally and systemically. There is one published report showing a relationship between formocresol pulpotomies in primary teeth and enamel defects in the permanent successors. These findings have not been confirmed in further studies.

Possible systemic toxicity was reported after 16 pulpotomies were carried out on one dog. However, there are no substantial data to support any toxic effects in humans—and, given the widespread use of formocresol for pulpotomies throughout the world since the 1930s and few reported ill-effects, there is no reason to doubt its safety.

Attempts have been made to find a suitable replacement for formocresol with little success. The following are among the medicaments that have been investigated.

Glutaraldehyde

Introduced by s'Gravenmade (1975) as a possible alternative to formocresol, glutaraldehyde has been extensively tested in vivo. It is theoretically a better fixative agent, having two functional aldehyde groups. However, success rates only comparable to those of formocresol have been reported by most investigators, including ourselves, and despite its reported advantages over formocresol, it has never found widespread use for pulpotomies in primary teeth. Recently, toxic properties of glutaraldehyde, such as allergic reactions and eye irritation, have come to light, and it is unlikely that it will replace formocresol as a medicament of choice for primary molar pulpotomies.

Calcium hydroxide

Calcium hydroxide, used extensively for permanent teeth, has been evaluated as a possible alternative to formocresol for primary teeth. The success rates reported for pulpotomies performed with calcium hydroxide have consistently been poor (around 60%) compared with those of formocresol, which are as high as 98% in some investigations. The most frequent cause of failure when calcium hydroxide is used is extensive internal resorption below the amputation site. *Its use in the pulp treatment of primary teeth is therefore contraindicated* at present.

Other experimental methods

The use of electrosurgery, CO_2 lasers, ferric sulphate and enriched collagen solution has been reported. These methods are, however, only at an experimental stage, and cannot be accepted for routine use in clinical practice.

The medicament of choice for pulpotomies in primary teeth at present remains formocresol, used as a 1/5 dilution of the original Buckley's formula.

B. THE PULPECTOMY TECHNIQUE

As discussed in Section A above, irreversible changes may occur very early in the dental pulp of the primary teeth. When the carious primary tooth is vital and the inflammation is confined to the coronal pulp tissue, pulpotomy is indicated and has a good prognosis. However, the inflammation is often found to extend to the radicular tissue, as is evident from uncontrollable haemorrhage even after the application of formocresol. Worse still, the tooth may be completely non-vital and an abscess may develop with or without acute cellulitis, a distressing complication. If this happens, many practitioners will often extract the tooth or at best perform a non-vital pulpotomy. The success rate of the latter procedure is poor, and in the authors' opinion it is obsolete and should not be carried out.

A pulpectomy procedure, which has been described in the paediatric dental literature for over 20 years, is the technique of choice. Pulpectomy is perhaps one of the most misunderstood techniques in paediatric dentistry. Many textbooks have described the pulp morphology of primary molars as complex, with many fine accessory root canals, which has led to the belief that a pulpectomy is difficult to perform. Nothing is further from the truth. It is true that some primary teeth do have a complex root morphology, but this does not contraindicate pulpectomy. This technique has been used successfully to retain non-vital and abscessed primary teeth for over two decades in the USA.

The aim of this section is to help in the understanding of the rationale, indications and limitations of this technique and to present a step-by-step clinical method for carrying it out in primary teeth.

Rationale for pulpectomy

The rationale for this technique is to gain access to the root canals, remove as much dead and infected material as possible and fill the root canals with a suitable material to maintain the primary tooth in a non-infected state.

Indications for pulpectomy

Irreversible inflammation extending to the radicular pulp

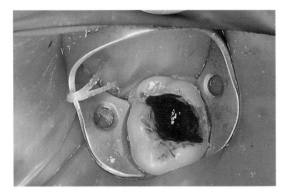

Figure 4.23 After removal of the coronal pulp, the haemorrhage from the root canal tissue should be pale red and easy to control. Extensive and persistent bleeding even after four minute application of formocresol implies irreversible inflammation of the radicular tissue, and is an indication for a pulpectomy.

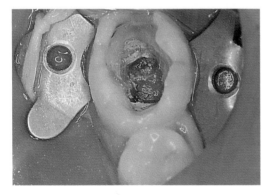

Primary teeth with necrotic pulps

Figure 4.24 Sometimes patients present with carious, asymptomatic primary teeth that, on accessing the pulp chamber, are found to be pulpless with necrotic pulps, as shown in the photograph. A pulpectomy should be carried out on such teeth.

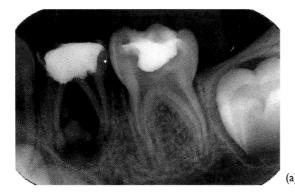

(a)

Primary teeth with evidence of furcation pathology

Figure 4.25 Infection in primary teeth usually manifests in the bi/trifurcation region, as opposed to the periapical pathology usually seen in permanent molars. This is because many fine channels of communication exist between the pulp chamber and the bone in the furcation area. (b) illustrates this point in an extracted primary molar. Note granulation tissue from the abscess in the bifurcation.

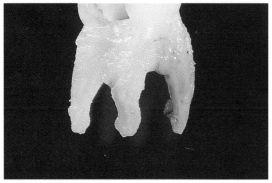

(b)

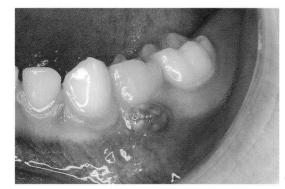

(a)

Presence of an abscess

Figure 4.26 The presence of a chronic, draining sinus (a) or an acute abscess with or without an associated cellulitis (b) is also an indication for a pulpectomy.

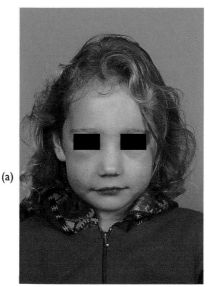

(b)

Contraindications

The medical contraindications for a pulpectomy are the same as those for a pulpotomy (see Section A). Other contraindications are as follows.

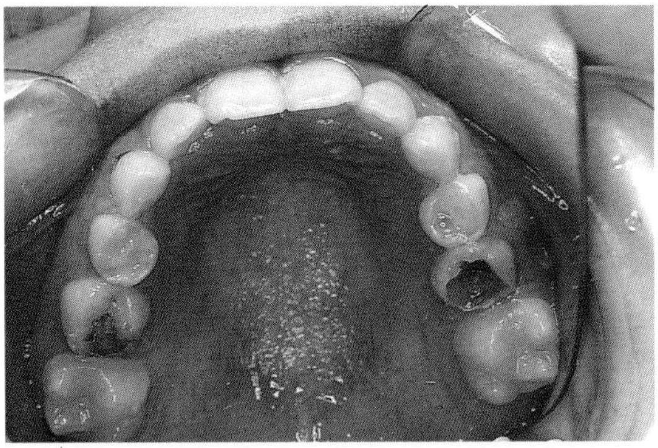

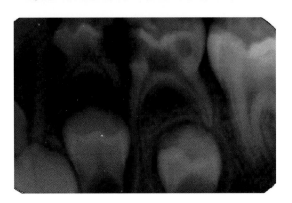

Unrestorable crown

Figure 4.27 A large lesion in 65. After removal of all caries, there will not be enough tooth structure left to support a stainless steel crown restoration, which would be required after a pulpectomy.

Advanced pathological root resorption

Figure 4.28 Peri-apical radiograph showing pathological root resorption due to a chronic abscess in 74. Extraction of this tooth rather than restoration is the treatment of choice.

Root canal filling material for pulpectomy in primary teeth

Any material that is used to fill the root canal of primary teeth must be capable of being totally resorbed at the same rate as the roots, when the primary tooth is being exfoliated. The most widely accepted and successful root canal filling material used for pulpectomies in primary teeth is pure zinc oxide and eugenol mixed as a slurry. Only pure zinc oxide and eugenol should be used, since this is entirely resorbable. If some of the paste is extruded through the apex, it will be completely resorbed by the periapical tissues (Figure 4.29). Recent research supports this observation. Proprietary brands of zinc oxide and eugenol (e.g. Kalzinol) may contain other ingredients, which may not be readily resorbable. In this case lumps of the filler paste may be left behind within the alveolar bone, causing a deviation in the path of eruption of the permanent successor.

The use of other root canal filling materials such as Maisto's paste and iodoform paste has been reported. However, pure zinc oxide and eugenol is still considered the best root canal filling material for primary teeth.

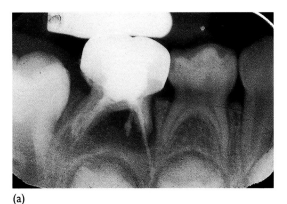

(a)

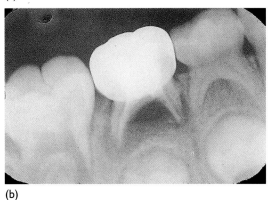

(b)

Figure 4.29 (a) Zinc oxide and eugenol is extruded through the apex of 85. (b) Three months later there is complete disappearance of the material from the peri-apical tissues.

Types of pulpectomy techniques

Pulpectomy can be accomplished in either one or two visits, depending upon the clinical signs and symptoms present. Two techniques will therefore be described:
* one-stage–single-visit pulpectomy;
* two-stage–two-visit pulpectomy.

One-stage–single-visit pulpectomy

Indications for single-visit pulpectomy

* Presence of inflamed but vital radicular pulp as shown in Figure 4.23.

* An asymptomatic primary tooth with necrotic pulp tissue (Figure 4.24) without any associated acute symptoms, such as cellulitis.
* Presence of a chronic buccal lesion without any active discharge or acute symptoms, such as shown in Figure 4.26a.

One-stage pulpectomy: step-by-step technique

In the one-stage–single-visit pulpectomy technique the complete restoration of the tooth is accomplished in a single visit. The root canals are located, filed, cleansed and filled with zinc oxide and eugenol, and the final restoration, usually a stainless steel crown, is placed in the same visit.

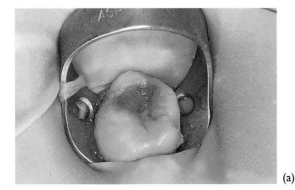

(a)

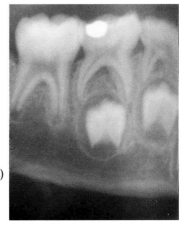

(b)

Step 1: Give local analgesia and isolate the tooth with rubber dam

Figure 4.30   (a) This shows 85 isolated with rubber dam. There was a history of occasional pain soon after the Ketac silver restoration was placed. A radiograph showed rarefaction in the bifurcation area, an indication for a pulpectomy (b). A pre-operative radiograph, usually a peri-apical, should always be taken.

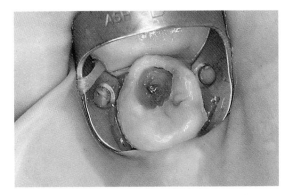

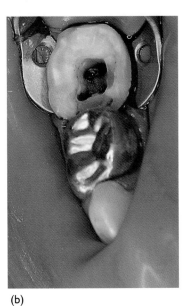

(a)

(b)

Step 2: Remove caries and identify exposure site

Figure 4.31 Following removal of old, failed restoration, showing point of exposure.

Step 3: Remove roof of pulp chamber as described for pulpotomy, and identify opening of root canals

Figure 4.32 Primary molars usually have the same number of root canals as permanent molars, namely three or four for lower molars and three for upper molars. (a) The opening of the mesiobuccal, mesiolingual and distal canals in 85. (b) Another lower molar (85) with four root canals, a second distal canal being present in this case. In most cases the root canals can be identified without much difficulty.

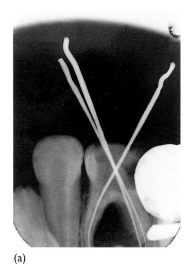

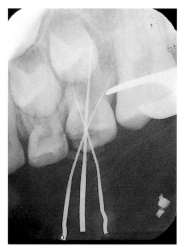

(a)

(b)

Step 4: Take a diagnostic radiograph with files in the root canals

Figure 4.33 This step is optional, and a diagnostic radiograph can be taken in a very cooperative child. In the authors' experience it is not usually required, and the rough length of the roots can be determined from the pre-operative radiograph. (a) Files in the mesial and distal canals of 74. (b) Files have been placed in the mesial, distal and palatal canals of 55.

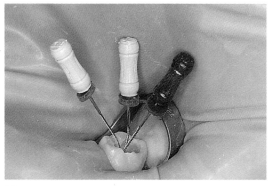

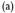

(a)

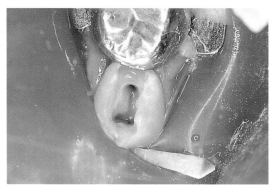

(b)

Step 5: Clean out root canals with Hedstrom files and remove remnants of pulp tissue and irrigate canals with saline

Figure 4.34 The root canals are filed to within 1–2 mm of the apex with Hedstrom files (a). Care is taken not to go beyond the apex in order to prevent any possible damage to the developing permanent successor. The root canals are filed lightly, since the roots of primary teeth are fragile and usually curved. Reaming is not advisable for the same reason. Any previous haemorrhage (b) should disappear at this stage (c). The root canals are filed to no more than size 30. Reproduced from *Dental Update* by permission of George Warman UK Ltd.

(c)

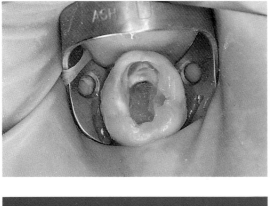

Step 6: Dry root canals with paper points and place a pledget of formocresol in the pulp chamber for four minutes

Figure 4.35 A pledget of formocresol is placed in the pulp chamber, after drying the root canals with absorbent paper points. Formocresol is used to 'fix' any tissue that may have been left behind in the apical 1–2 mm of the root canals and in any accessory canals that may be present.

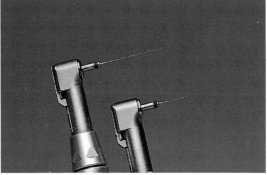

Step 7: Select a spiral root canal filler of appropriate size

Figure 4.36 A spiral root canal filler, one size smaller than the last file used in the root canals, should be used to fill the root canals. This is to prevent it from engaging and fracturing in the root canal. Using sharp scissors, the spiral filler is cut to half its length. which makes it easier to handle in a child's mouth and also prevents the filling material from being pushed through the apex.

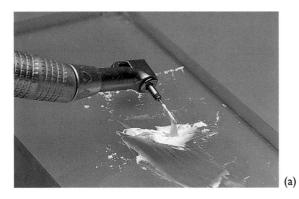

(a)

Step 8: Mix zinc oxide and eugenol as a slurry, and spin it into the root canals using the spiral root canal filler

Figure 4.37 Pure zinc oxide and eugenol are mixed into a slurry. This is then carried into the root canals with the spiral root canal filler (a) and spun into the root canals (b). If the clinician is not familiar with the spiral fillers, it is advisable that the zinc oxide and eugenol be carried into the root canals with either a Hedstrom file or a fine guttapercha point and agitated a few times to ensure adequate filling of the canals.

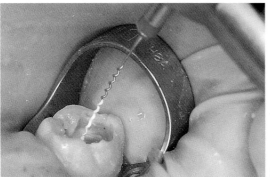

(b)

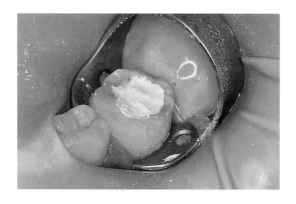

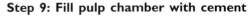

Step 9: Fill pulp chamber with cement

Figure 4.38 The pulp chamber is filled with one of the proprietary brands of zinc oxide and eugenol cements such as Kalzinol.

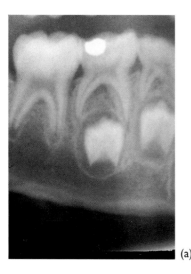

Step 10: Restore the tooth with a stainless steel crown

Figure 4.39 The 85 treated with a pulpectomy and restored with a stainless steel crown.

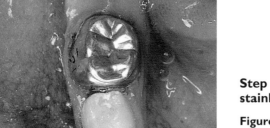

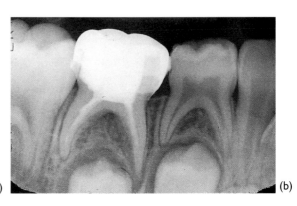

(a)   (b)

Step 11: Take a postoperative radiograph to check root filling

Figure 4.40 Pre- (a) and post- (b) operative radiographs of the case shown above. Note that the root canals are filled adequately and short of the apex. This is desirable, but may not always be achieved.

Follow-up

Teeth that have been treated with the pulpectomy technique should be reviewed both clinically and radiographically at follow-up appointments. The pulpectomy is judged to be clinically successful if there is alleviation of acute symptoms and the tooth is free from pain and mobility. Any draining sinus should have disappeared.

The radiographic schedule that we recommend is one peri-apical radiograph taken pre-operatively, one immediately post-operative, and then at six months and 1 year later. The radiographs should be assessed for furcation pathology. An improvement of the bone condition in the furcation region as shown in Figure 4.41, or no further deterioration in the condition of that region, means that the pulpectomy has been successful. Any worsening of the extent of the radiolucency in the furcation region is an indication for extraction of the tooth.

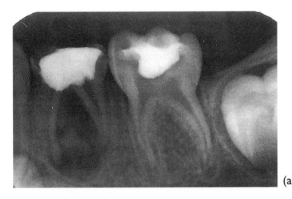

(a)

Figure 4.41 Pre, post and follow-up radiographs of an abscessed 74 successfully treated with a pulpectomy technique: (a) pre-operative radiograph showing an abscess on 74 causing destruction of the bone, typically in the furcation area; (b) post-operative radiograph showing root canal filling in place; (c) radiograph six months later showing resolution of radiolucent area on 75 shown in (a). Reproduced from *Dental Update* by permission of George Warman UK Ltd.

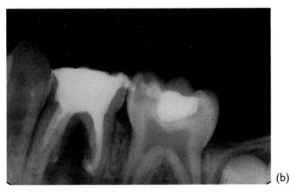

(b)

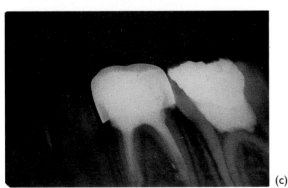

(c)

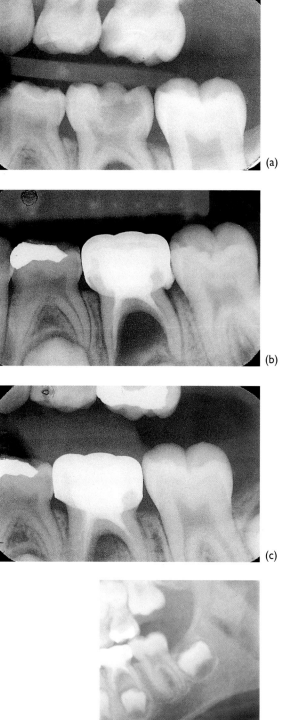

(a)

(b)

(c)

(d)

Other examples of root fillings in primary molars

Case 1

Figure 4.42 Serial radiographs showing gradual regeneration of bone in the bifurcation area after a pulpectomy was performed on 75: (a) pre-operative; (b) immediately post-operative; (c) three months later; (d) one year later.

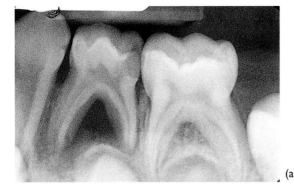

(a)

Case 2

Figure 4.43 Serial radiographs showing a successful pulpectomy performed on 74 indicating a continuous improvement of bone in the bifurcation over a six month period: (a) pre-operative; (b) six months later.

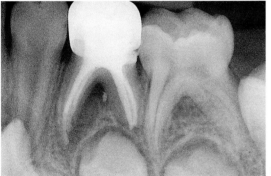

(b)

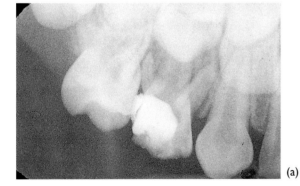

(a)

Case 3

Figure 4.44 An example of a pulpectomy performed in an upper molar (54): (a) pre-operative; (b) post-operative. Note the filling in the mesial, distal and palatal canals.

(b)

Is a spiral root filler the best instrument for root filling?

A recent study has shown that the spiral root canal filler may be the best instrument for this technique. An added advantage of this instrument is that it may also spin the zinc oxide and eugenol paste into the accessory canals, which can be present in primary molars, as seen frequently in postoperative radiographs (Figure 4.45). The spiral root filler is a fragile instrument, and if not used carefully can fracture in the root canal (Figure 4.46).

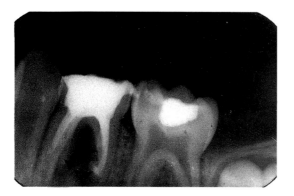

Figure 4.45 Peri-apical radiograph of a root-filled primary molar (74) showing evidence of root filling material in an accessory canal marked with arrows.

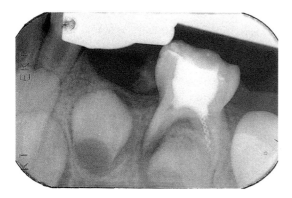

Figure 4.46 A spiral root filler fractured in the distal canal of 75.

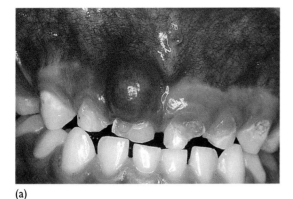

(a)

Figure 4.47 An abscessed primary incisor (51) treated with a pulpectomy technique: (a) pre-operative view showing abscess in relation to 51; (b) peri-apical radiograph showing apical radiolucent area; (c) root filling in place.

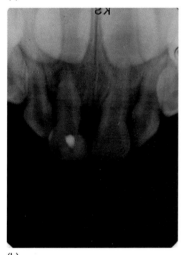

(b)

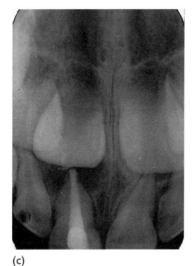

(c)

Two-stage–two-visit pulpectomy

The indications for a two-stage pulpectomy are:

- presence of an acute abscess with or without associated cellulitis, as shown in Figure 4.26(b);
- presence of active and persistent discharge from the root canals.

The two-stage pulpectomy technique

Stage I/Visit I: Emergency management of the acute abscess

When an acute abscess is present, it must be resolved as quickly as possible. This is achieved either by gaining drainage through the carious cavity or, if a fistula is present, by puncturing it to improve drainage (usually a painless procedure). Local analgesia should be used if possible because it is a common clinical finding to encounter vital pulp tissue in an infected pulp chamber (Figure 4.34b). Root canals are identified, lightly filed to drain as much of the abscess as possible, and also irrigated. A pledget of formocresol is then sealed in the pulp chamber with a suitable cement. Antibiotics should be prescribed in the presence of an acute infection with associated cellulitis, or other systemic symptoms. Our own research has shown that the use of a two-dose regimen of amoxycillin allows a pulpectomy to be carried out as early as 48 hours after the initial drainage.

Stage 2/Visit 2: Final root canal filling

The patient is recalled seven to ten days later. At this stage, the tooth should be free from clinical symptoms, and any abscess should have resolved or be resolving. The tooth should be opened under rubber dam, root canals accessed and the pulpectomy procedure completed as described before.

Pulpectomy for abscessed primary incisors (Figure 4.47)

Non-vital or abscessed primary incisors can also be treated with a pulpectomy technique in the same way as described previously for primary molars.

Reported success rates for primary tooth pulpectomies

Most investigators have reported high success rates—over 80% for pulpectomies performed in primary teeth.

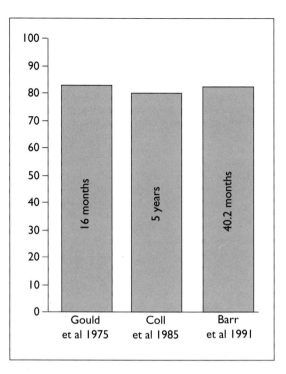

Figure 4.48 Histogram showing reported success rates for single-visit pulpectomies with follow-up periods ranging from 16 months to five years.

5 Stainless Steel Crowns for Primary Molars

The nickel chrome crown—commonly called the stainless steel crown—has proved to be the most successful restoration for large cavities in primary teeth (Figure 5.1). Following the treatment of pulpally involved teeth, a restoration is required that will satisfy several criteria. Ideally it should have the same lifespan as that remaining for the tooth and should provide protection to the remaining tooth structure that has been rendered weak and brittle after the pulp therapy. Several studies have examined the lifespan of amalgam restorations in primary teeth and found that a significant number need to be replaced within the lifespan of the teeth. Our research has shown that, once fitted, stainless steel crowns rarely need to be replaced. In contrast, amalgams, composites and glass ionomer cements must often be replaced, except in those cases where they have been used for the restoration of small one- or two-surface cavities. In addition to providing full coverage of teeth weakened by large removal of tooth substance, stainless steel crowns also provide protection from future carious attack in those teeth, especially in 'high-caries-risk' children who are prone to developing new and secondary lesions.

The technique of placing a stainless steel restoration is simple, and in the hands of most clinicians can be performed far faster than a multi-surface restoration with other materials. Modern crowns are so well constructed that extensive trimming and adjustments prior to fitting are not usually required, and tooth preparation is minimal and quick. Preformed and precrimped stainless steel crowns are widely available in the United Kingdom and throughout Europe (3M Dental, Loughborough, UK). Once experience has been gained, two adjacent crowns in the same quadrants can be placed in less than 20 minutes. One of the greatest advantages is that the failure rate is very low, and is far better than that reported for any other type of restoration in primary molars.

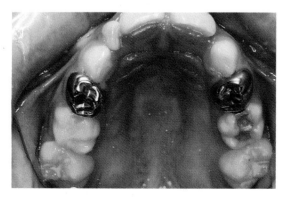

Figure 5.1 This shows 54 and 64 restored with stainless steel crowns.

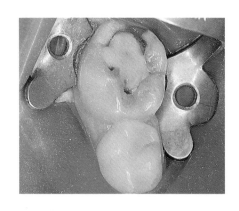

Indications for stainless steel crowns

Restoration of primary molars requiring large multisurface restoration

Figure 5.2 A failed disto-occlusal composite restoration placed in 85. Such large cavities are best restored with stainless steel crowns.

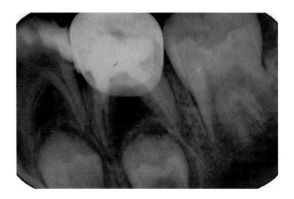

Restoration of teeth in children with rampant caries

Figure 5.3 Because these children are prone to secondary caries, stainless steel crown restorations afford protection by virtue of the full coverage that they provide.

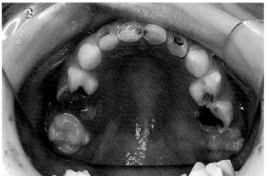

Restoration of teeth after pulp therapy

Figure 5.4 After pulp therapy, primary molars are usually more brittle and prone to fracture. A stainless steel restoration should always be placed on teeth treated with pulp therapy. The photograph shows 75 restored with a stainless steel crown after a pulpectomy.

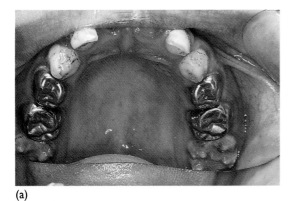

(a)

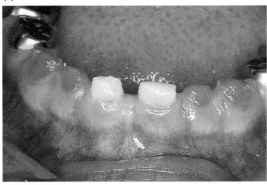

(b)

Restoration of teeth with developmental defects

Figure 5.5 (a) Primary molars of a patient with hypomineralized amelogenesis imperfecta restored with stainless steel crowns. (b) Similar restorations placed in a patient with dentinogenesis imperfecta.

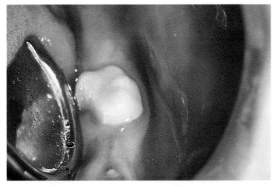

Restoration of fractured primary molars

Figure 5.6 This shows 75 with a fractured mesio-lingual cusp. A stainless steel crown is indicated.

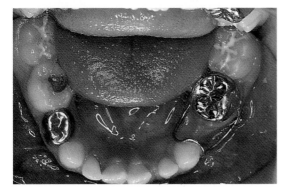

As an abutment for space maintainers

Figure 5.7 Intra-oral photograph of a patient who needed a stainless steel crown on 75 and extraction of 74. A band and loop space maintainer was indicated, and was soldered to the crown placed on 75. An impression was first taken with the crown placed on 75 but not cemented. After removal from the tooth and placing in the impression, it was sent to the laboratory, where a loop was soldered to it.

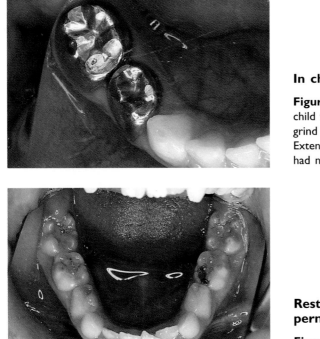

In children with bruxism

Figure 5.8 Stainless steel crowns placed in a young child with bruxism. Note that the child had started to grind through the crowns one year after placement. Extensive attrition would have resulted if the crowns had not been placed.

(a)

Restoration of hypoplastic young permanent molars

Figure 5.9 Hypoplastic 36 and 46 (a) restored with stainless steel crowns (b).

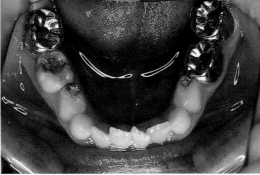

(b)

Armamentarium

The stainless steel crowns available in the UK and Europe are manufactured by 3M Dental. They come in several sizes, numbered from 2 to 7 (Figure 5.10).

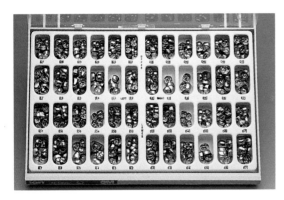

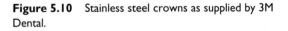

Figure 5.10   Stainless steel crowns as supplied by 3M Dental.

Other special equipment that is required is shown in Figure 5.11.

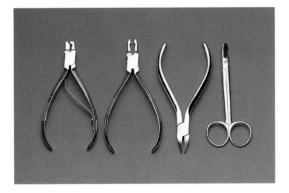

Figure 5.11   Pliers (Johnson 114) and crimping pliers (Unitek 800-108) are needed, although in our experience Adams pliers, readily available in most practices are adequate for crimping the crown margins. Crown cutting scissors, again available in most practices, are also required.

Step-by-step technique for fitting stainless steel crowns

The preparation of the tooth is carried out in several steps. While the order described here is not crucial, it is a useful guide for students and practitioners fitting stainless steel crowns for the first time.

Step 1: Local analgesia and rubber dam

Local analgesia should be administered, although it may not always be necessary when preparing a tooth that has undergone pulp therapy. Nevertheless, even in these teeth there will need to be some preparation involving the gingival margin, which can cause some discomfort. Rubber dam should also be used. Because the preparation for a crown is usually carried out at the same visit as the pulp therapy, local analgesia and rubber dam are already in place. When

the stainless steel crown is fitted for extensive caries or for some other reason, rubber dam is required. Wherever possible, the rubber dam clamp should be placed on the tooth distal to the one being restored. However, difficulty arises if the tooth that needs clamping is the tooth being prepared for the crown (Figure 5.12), the proximal reduction distally becoming difficult because the bur will be caught in the rubber dam sheet. In these instances it is recommended that all necessary reduction, except the distal proximal slice, be carried out under rubber dam. The dam is then removed, the distal slice completed and the crown fitted without the dam. Alternatively, the rubber dam can be held clear of the distal surface by the dental surgery assistant with a flat plastic instrument while the distal surface is being reduced as shown in Figure 5.31. Note in Figure 5.12 that the rubber dam is placed using the trough method, described in Chapter 3, which gives access to the mesial surface for reduction.

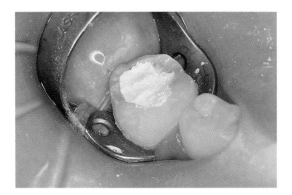

Figure 5.12   This shows 85 isolated with rubber dam, using the trough technique. This allows access to the mesial surface for reduction after occlusal reduction is complete.

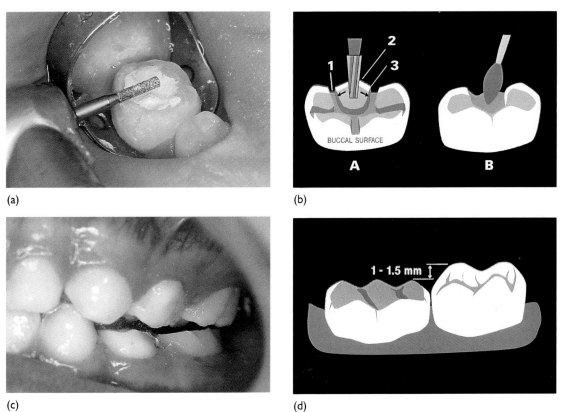

(a)

(b)

(c)

(d)

Step 2: Reduction of occlusal height

Figure 5.13 This is done using either a large flat diamond bur (a) or a diamond stone. To reduce cusps, for those who are still learning the use of stainless steel crowns, it is advisable to cut a groove into the fissures of the teeth with a suitable bur and then reduce the height of the crown to that level. This is illustrated in (b): A – carbide bur used to reduce cusps: 1, reduced grooves; 2, cusp tip; 3, cusp slope. B – diamond bur used to reduce cusps. Once experience has been gained, following the occlusal anatomy the crown is reduced until the tooth is completely out of occlusion and there is room to fit the crown (c). If a rubber dam is used, it is difficult to check the occlusion. A useful guide in these cases is the occlusal table of the adjacent teeth as seen in the example of the completed occlusal reduction on the mandibular left second primary molar (d).

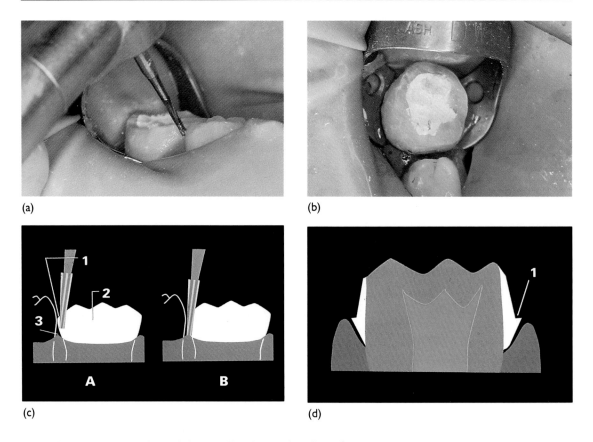

(a)   (b)

(c)   (d)

Step 3: Reduction of mesial and distal proximal surfaces

Figure 5.14 A tapered tungsten carbide (a) or tapered diamond bur is swept bucco-lingually through the mesial (b) and distal contact points to ensure sufficient clearance for the seating of the crown. Great care is taken to avoid accidentally removing the enamel from the adjacent tooth. The best precaution is either to place a wooden wedge between teeth before the proximal reduction is attempted or to ensure that there is some tooth structure proximal to the bur when it is being moved bucco-lingually as seen on the diagrams of the proximal slice (c): A – starting the proximal slice (bur moved to lingual): 1, tooth structure visible proximal to bur; 2, buccal surface; 3, gingival crest. B – completing proximal slice (bur swept bucco-lingually). The proximal reduction is the most crucial part of the preparation, and close attention must be paid to ensure that no gingival step or ledge (d,1) exists; this would prevent seating of the crown. Bleeding from the interdental papilla is inevitable, and should not deter the operator from extending the preparation gingivally to remove a ledge. When the mesial/distal reduction is complete, a check is made with a probe that no step exists and there is ample clearance for the crown.

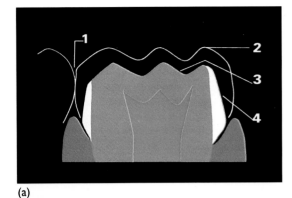

(a)

(b)

Step 4: Round-off sharp edges and make a final check of the preparation

Figure 5.15 The sharp edges of enamel are rounded-off and the preparation finally checked for accuracy. There should be adequate occlusal and proximal clearance without any ledges proximally as seen on the mesial-distal section of the prepared tooth (a): 1, contact broken; 2, structure removed; 3, occlusal reduction; 4, proximal reduction. (b) The completed preparation of 85.

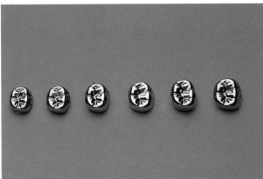

(a)

(b)

Step 5: Select a crown for a trial fit

Figure 5.16 With experience, an estimate can be made of the probable size of the crown that is most likely to fit. To begin with, it is advisable to first measure the mesio-distal width of the tooth with calipers prior to preparation, and use this to select a crown of appropriate size. Different sizes, ranging from 2 to 7, are available (a), and can be tried until one fits. It is usually better to first seat the crown lingually and then rotate it buccally as demonstrated in (b): 1, rounded bevel; 2, buccal surface; 3, lingual surface. The crown should snap onto the tooth with little pressure. If the crown does not fit with a 'snap' then usually it is too big and a smaller size should be tried.

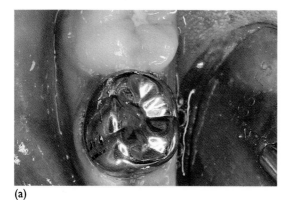

(a)

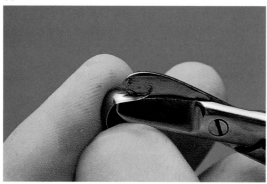

(b)

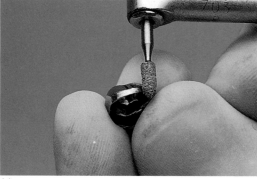

(c)

Step 6: Adjust the crown if required

Figure 5.17 Modern crowns are well constructed and usually do not require adjustment. However, occasionally the crown margins may need to be trimmed if there is blanching of the marginal gingivae when the crown is fully seated (a). Some blanching will always occur, and is acceptable. If there is excessive blanching then the crown margins can be trimmed using sharp crown cutting scissors (b). If this is done, a green stone is always used around the margins of the crown to smooth and remove any sharp edges (c).

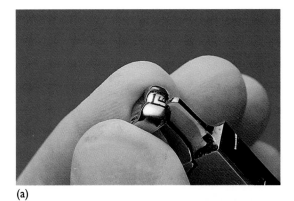

(a)

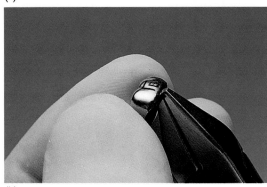

(b)

Step 7: Crimp the crown margins

Figure 5.18 The crown margins are crimped with either the crimping pliers (a) or with an Adams plier (b). The aim of this step is to ensure good adaptation of the crown margins to the tooth, to give a tight fit and to prevent build-up of plaque on the crown. (c) Crown margins before crimping. (d) Crown margins after crimping.

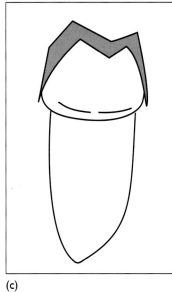

(c)

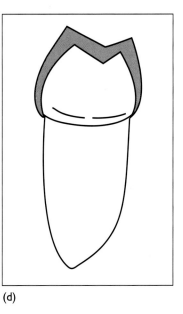

(d)

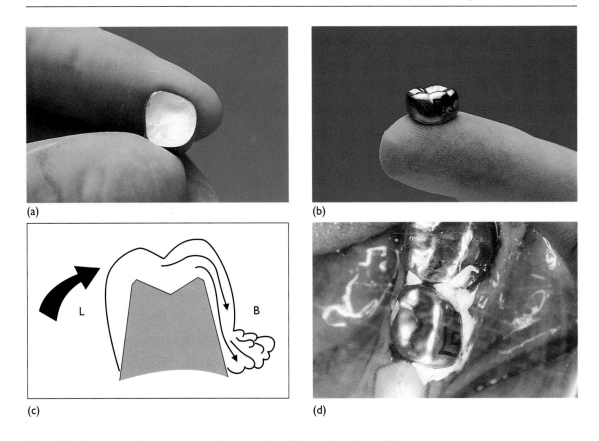

(a)   (b)

(c)   (d)

Step 8: Cement the crown on the tooth with polycarboxylate cement

Figure 5.19 The crown should be filled with a polycarboxylate cement, such as Poly-F. It is important that sufficient cement be mixed, to almost fill the crown (a). The crown should be handed to the dentist, full of cement,
on the fingertip (b) so that the dentist can see the crown form and hence the orientation for cementing. The crown
is seated onto the tooth on the lingual side (L) first, and then pushed over onto the buccal (B) side (c). If properly
adapted and crimped, there should be a resistance to seating followed by a snap as the crown fits into place. If a
rubber dam is being used, pressure is applied by the dentist to the crown while the cement sets. If a rubber dam
is not being used, or has been removed prior to cementation, then the child can be instructed to bite the teeth
together. If two adjacent teeth are being crowned at the same visit then both crowns are seated at the same time
(d).

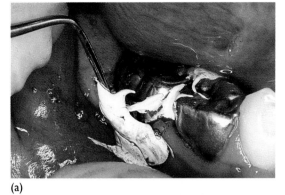
(a)

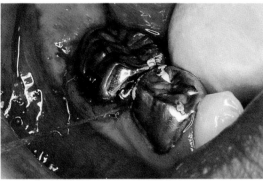
(b)

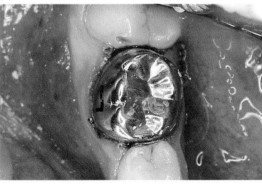
(a)

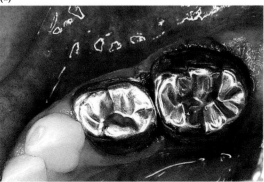
(b)

Step 9: Remove excess cement

Figure 5.20 Allow the cement to set, when any excess can be easily flaked away with a suitable instrument (a). It is important to ensure that no excess cement is left at the mesial and distal gingival margins of the crown. This is best accomplished by taking a piece of dental floss and tying a single knot in it. This is then passed backwards and forwards through the gingival embrasure, removing any excess cement (b). A rubber cup and pumice prophylaxis is useful to finally polish the crowns.

Step 10: Make a final check of completed restoration

Figure 5.21 Finally, the crown should be checked for occlusion and lightly polished with a prophylaxis paste. Any minor discrepancies in the occlusion should be ignored, since once crowned, the primary molars seem to be able to adjust themselves very quickly. (a) Completed restoration on 85. (b) Completed restorations of 84 and 85 accomplished in the same visit. (c) Diagrammatic representation of the completed restoration in bucco-lingual section: 1, occlusal surface of crown; 2, occlusal preparation; 3, cement; 4, adaptation to natural bulge; 5, gingival margin, 6, adaptation to natural undercut.

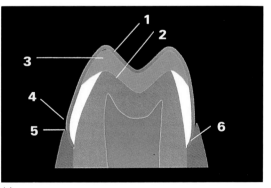
(c)

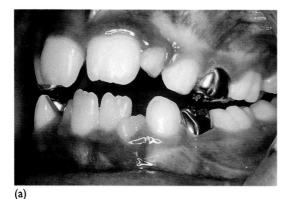

(a)

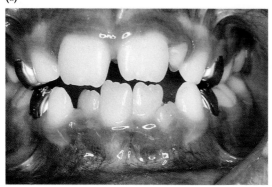

(b)

Follow-up

Figure 5.22 (a, b) At each recall appointment the crowns should be checked for occlusion, fit and seating. Particular attention should be given to the condition of the gingival margins around the crowns. Well adapted and crimped margins facilitate plaque removal with routine oral hygiene measures. The photographs show excellent gingival health around well adapted crowns on primary molars.

Some problems and their solution

Crown does not seat proximally

This usually means that there is a ledge, as discussed before. It is removed using a tapered fissure bur.

Loss of space

Sometimes loss of space has occurred because of proximal caries in the tooth being restored and movement of the tooth distal to it into the space. In this situation a stainless steel crown that will fit on the tooth bucco-lingually is too large mesio-distally. There are two possible solutions to this problem: Figures 5.23 and 5.24.

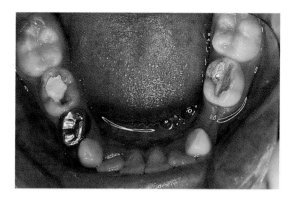

Figure 5.23 The crown is rotated slightly mesio-buccally so that it is rotated slightly out of the arch.

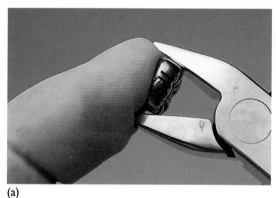

(a)

Figure 5.24 The closest fitting crown is held in the beaks of the Adams plier (a) and squeezed mesio-distally to reduce this dimension. This is an effective way of flattening the contact points (b) and reducing the crown mesio-distally, but careful crimping of the crown margins is required later because the crown margins will be distorted by this method.

(b)

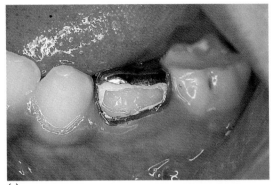

(a)

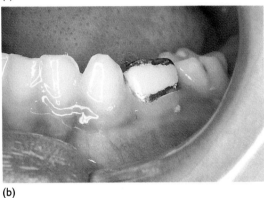

(b)

Parents' concern about aesthetics

Figure 5.25 Parents rarely object to the placement of stainless steel crowns. However, if they are concerned about this aspect, the crowns can be made more aesthetic by cutting a window in the buccal aspect (a) and placing a composite resin facing (b).

Concerns about exfoliation

Stainless steel crowns do not interfere in any way with the normal exfoliation of the primary molars, with the stainless steel crown and the primary molar crown being exfoliated together (Figure 5.26).

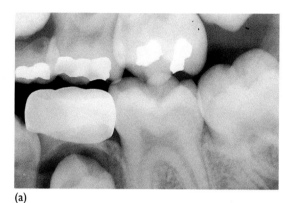

(a)

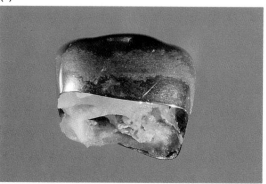

(b)

Figure 5.26 (a) Radiograph showing normal resorption of 75 restored with a stainless steel crown. (b) Normal exfoliation of the molar shown in (a). (c) The exfoliated 75. This is the norm rather than an exception.

(c)

Success rates of stainless steel crowns compared with other restorations in primary molars

Recent research has shown that stainless steel crown restoration of primary molars is superior to that achieved with amalgam, composite resin or glass ionomer cement. Once fitted, the crowns seldom need replacing. Our own research has shown that five years after placement over 80% of stainless steel crowns are still in place (Figure 1.9).

In paediatric dentistry only those techniques that need to be performed once in the lifetime of the primary tooth are justified. Repeated replacement of restorations in children is traumatic and can put the child off future dental treatment. In view of the reported superiority of the stainless

steel crown for the restoration of large cavities in primary molars, all clinicians who treat children should be familiar with this technique.

Completing both pulpotomy and stainless steel crown in the same visit

Efforts should be made to complete both pulpotomy and stainless steel crowns in the same visit, under rubber dam. This will reduce the number of times the child requires the administration of local analgesia. The following sequence (Figures 5.27–5.36) shows how this can be accomplished in the shortest possible time.

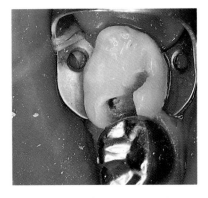

Figure 5.27 Remove caries and identify exposure as discussed in Chapter 4.

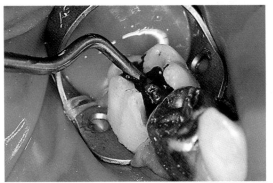

Figure 5.28 Amputate coronal pulp using a large spoon excavator as shown or a large round bur with a slow-speed handpiece.

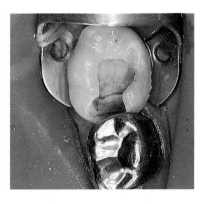

Figure 5.29 Place formocresol pledget in the pulp chamber.

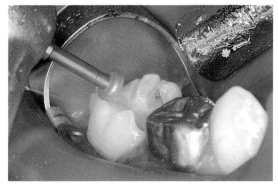

Figure 5.30 While the formocresol pledget is in place, a stainless steel crown preparation is started. The four minutes during which the formocresol must be applied to the pulp tissue is enough to complete a stainless steel crown preparation. Occlusal reduction is shown here being performed with a diamond wheel.

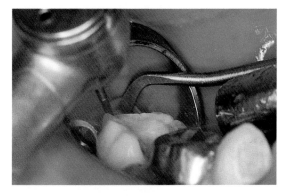

Figure 5.31 The mesial and distal reduction is carried out as described earlier in the chapter. The distal reduction can be accomplished by slipping a flat plastic instrument under the edge of the rubber dam sheet and pulling it away from the distal surface of the tooth.

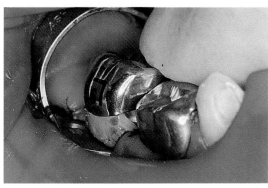

Figure 5.32 A stainless steel crown is selected and tried on the tooth, and any necessary adjustments are carried out.

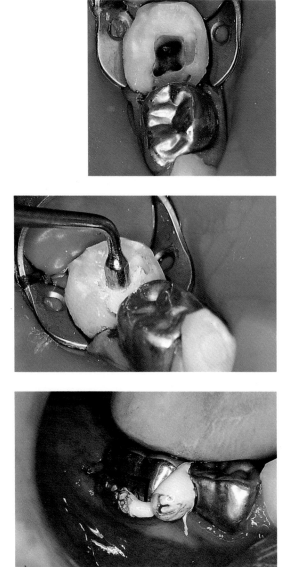

Figure 5.33 The formocresol pledget is now removed. Haemorrhage from the radicular tissue should have stopped.

Figure 5.34 The pulp chamber is filled with a cement, such as zinc oxide and eugenol.

Figure 5.35 The rubber dam is now removed and the crown full of cement is seated on the tooth.

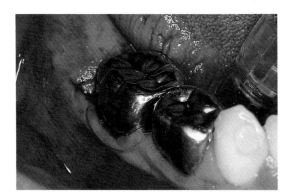

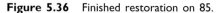

Figure 5.36 Finished restoration on 85.

6   Strip Crowns for Primary Incisors

Introduction

Unsightly or discoloured primary incisor teeth will often be the reason why, for the first time, parents seek dental treatment for their children. Such teeth may be carious, discoloured due to a congenital defect or trauma, or simply malformed. Caries of upper primary incisors is a consistent feature of 'nursing caries syndrome' (also known as 'nursing bottle caries' or 'bottle mouth caries'), and will often need restoration. Nursing caries is seen in pre-school children and results from frequent or prolonged consumption of fluids containing fermentable carbohydrate from a bottle or feeder cup. Fruit-based infant drinks are most commonly involved, but similar patterns of caries can also be seen with milk-based drinks and in infants breast-fed on demand. Such infants are often allowed to suck on the bottle as a pacifier throughout the night. During sleep, there is a considerable reduction in salivary flow rate, and consequently salivary buffering and mechanical cleansing are reduced to minimal levels. This results in rapid demineralization and clinically rampant caries. Typically, the maxillary incisors and first primary molars are most severely affected. The lower incisors are rarely affected, since they are protected during suckling by the tongue and directly bathed in secretions from the submandibular and sublingual glands.

The treatment of decayed primary incisors depends upon the stage of decay and the age and cooperation of the child patient. There are several options available to the dentist in treating such teeth. First and foremost, a comprehensive preventive programme, including dietary counselling, oral hygiene instruction and appropriate use of topical and systemic fluorides, is essential to arrest the caries process and prevent any further destruction (Chapter 1). In the past, interproximal discing of the teeth to render them

self-cleansing has been described, although this technique does not remove the decay nor is it aesthetically pleasing. Others have advocated the use of orthodontic bands, open-faced stainless steel crowns, acrylic crowns or polycarbonate crowns. In this chapter a method is described for the aesthetic restoration of primary incisors utilizing preformed celluloid crown forms specially produced for primary incisors to produce a mouth-formed, direct, full-coverage composite resin restoration. This is known as the 'strip crown technique'. Decayed, discoloured or malformed primary incisors may be restored using this method.

Indications for strip crowns

- Extensive or multisurface caries in primary incisors
- Congenitally malformed primary incisors
- Discoloured primary incisors discoloured following trauma
- Fractured primary incisors following trauma
- Congenitally discoloured primary incisors (e.g. through congenital erythropoietic porphyria)
- Amelogenesis imperfecta

Materials

Most materials required in this technique will be readily available in any dental surgery. These include standard restorative dental instruments, handpieces, a tapered high-speed bur, a small slow-speed round bur for caries removal, calcium hydroxide or glass ionomer lining cement, a light-cured composite with appropriate etchant and bonding agents, visible curing light and fine curved scissors. The celluloid crown forms are marketed as the 3M Strip Crown Kit (3M Dental, Loughborough, UK). This provides a range of sizes of crowns specifically designed and made for upper primary incisors.

Most modern hybrid or microfilled composite resin restorative systems can be used for the strip crown technique. However, there are several factors that should be taken into account when choosing materials if the best results are to be attained.

Several composite systems now include dentine shades that are more opaque than standard anterior composite. These are particularly useful, since they more effectively mask any residual discolouration of the underlying dentine or the whiteness of lining materials. In addition, encapsulated presentation is to be preferred, since it allows easy filling of the crown form.

Where little enamel remains following removal of caries, bonding of composite resin to both dentine and enamel is important for retention of the final restoration. Two bonding systems that will bond to dentine micromechanically are presently available. These are either resin-based (such as Gluma 2000) or solvent-based (such as ABC). Either are suitable for the strip crown technique.

Figures 6.1–6.24 show the preparation of four maxillary incisors—but of course a single tooth may be restored on its own. If it is proposed to restore all four maxillary incisors, this is best accomplished in one visit. However, if restoration over two visits is planned, it is advisable to restore the two central incisors at one and the two lateral incisors at the second. This allows for more accurate matching of colour and shape between left and right sides.

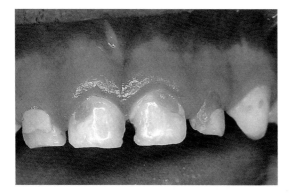

Figure 6.1 The teeth should be anaesthetized, if necessary, and then isolated. Cotton wool roll isolation is usually sufficient, although rubber dam or dry dam may be used if preferred.

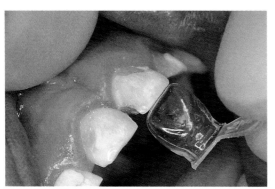

Figure 6.2 The size of the celluloid crown form is chosen. This may be accomplished by measuring the mesio-distal dimension of the space available with calipers and then checked by holding the form up to the incisal edge of the tooth.

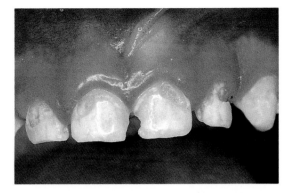

Figure 6.3 All caries is removed using a small round bur in a slow-speed handpiece.

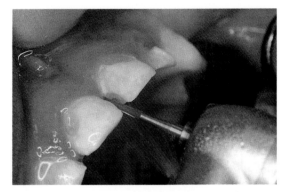

Figure 6.4 The teeth are then prepared for the strip crown. Using a tapered diamond or tungsten carbide bur in a high-speed handpiece, the length of the crown is reduced incisally. Mesial and distal slices are made, tapered to a knife edge at the gingival margin.

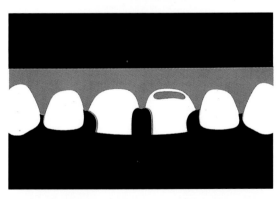

Figure 6.5 Diagram illustrating the mesial and distal walls of incisors prepared for strip crowns. The caries have been removed.

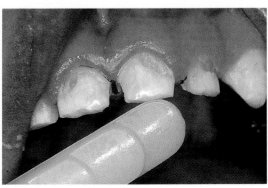

Figure 6.6 The shade of composite resin is chosen. When the tooth is discoloured, an adjacent tooth or the lower incisors can be used for shade matching.

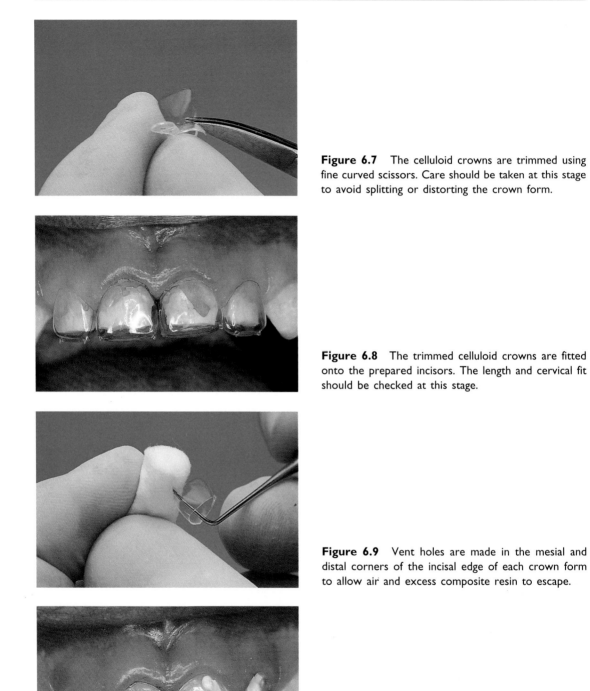

Figure 6.7 The celluloid crowns are trimmed using fine curved scissors. Care should be taken at this stage to avoid splitting or distorting the crown form.

Figure 6.8 The trimmed celluloid crowns are fitted onto the prepared incisors. The length and cervical fit should be checked at this stage.

Figure 6.9 Vent holes are made in the mesial and distal corners of the incisal edge of each crown form to allow air and excess composite resin to escape.

Figure 6.10 A proprietary calcium hydroxide paste or glass ionomer cement is applied to the pulpal wall of any exposed dentine.

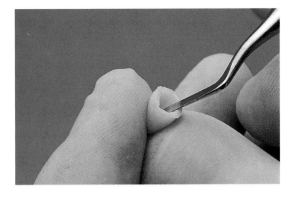

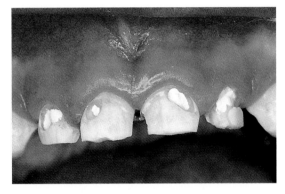

Figure 6.11 Composite resin is squeezed into the crown form and hollowed out in the centre to reduce the amount of excess.

Figure 6.12 The teeth are etched for one minute with a proprietary etchant, washed and dried. The opaque, frosty appearance of the enamel is evident in the illustration.

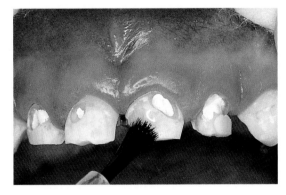

Figure 6.13 The bonding agent is applied, and then cured for 15 seconds, if applicable, according to the manufacturer's instructions.

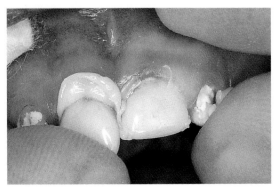

Figure 6.14 The crown forms, containing composite resin, are firmly seated on the prepared teeth. Again, care should be taken at this stage, since excess pressure can result in splitting of the crown form.

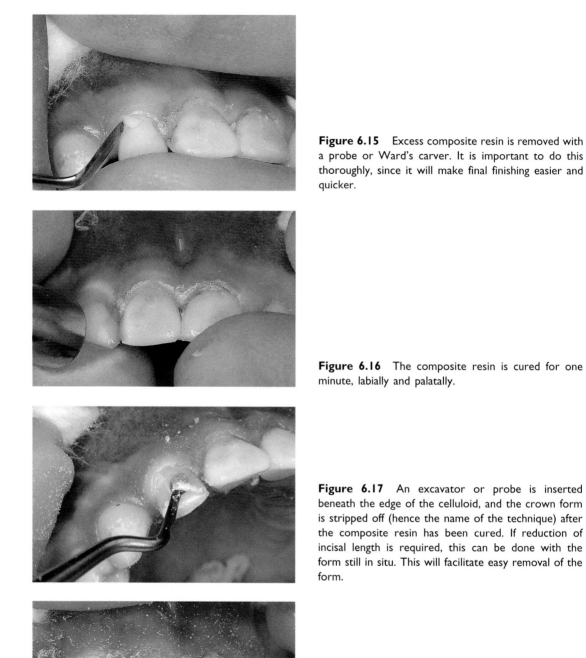

Figure 6.15 Excess composite resin is removed with a probe or Ward's carver. It is important to do this thoroughly, since it will make final finishing easier and quicker.

Figure 6.16 The composite resin is cured for one minute, labially and palatally.

Figure 6.17 An excavator or probe is inserted beneath the edge of the celluloid, and the crown form is stripped off (hence the name of the technique) after the composite resin has been cured. If reduction of incisal length is required, this can be done with the form still in situ. This will facilitate easy removal of the form.

Figure 6.18 The last step is to smooth and polish the crowns, although finishing is usually minimal. Flexible carborundum (Soflex, 3M Dental) discs are ideal for this, although fine diamond or Baker Curson high-speed burs may be preferred.

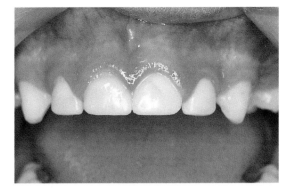

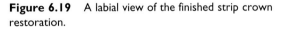

Figure 6.19 A labial view of the finished strip crown restoration.

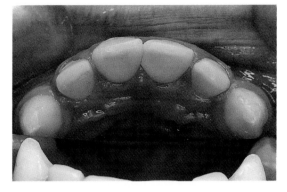

Figure 6.20 A palatal view of the finished strip crown restoration clearly demonstrating the full coverage provided by this restoration technique.

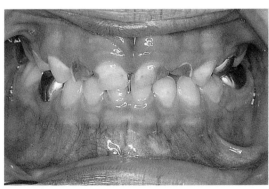

Figure 6.21 Pre-operative photograph of extensive caries of primary maxillary incisors.

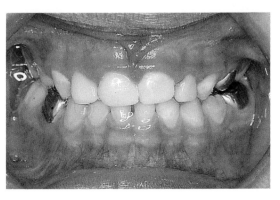

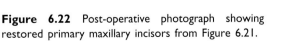

Figure 6.22 Post-operative photograph showing restored primary maxillary incisors from Figure 6.21.

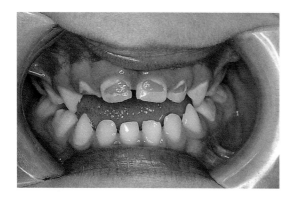

Figure 6.23 Pre-operative photograph of extensive caries of primary maxillary incisors.

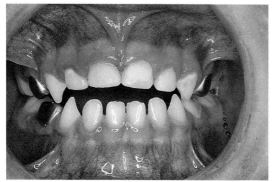

Figure 6.24 Post-operative photograph showing restored primary maxillary incisors from Figure 6.23.

Discussion

The strip crown technique is a quick, simple and effective method for the restoration of primary incisors. Most children are delighted by the improvement in their appearance, and it is hoped that this will encourage an interest in their dental health from both parents and child. Nevertheless, there are a few problems that might be encountered by the dentist. Some of these and their solutions are outlined in Table 6.1.

Table 6.1
Problems and solutions that may be encountered when using strip crowns

Problem	Solution
Tearing of celluloid crown form when trimming	Keep scissors exclusively for strip crown preparation
Splitting of filled crown form when seating it	Hollow out composite to reduce excess and use gentle pressure. A slow 'rocking' motion while seating the form helps excess composite to escape
Difficulty in stripping off crown form	Remove excess composite from gingival margin before curing
Calcium hydroxide showing through composite	If this is anticipated, a glass ionomer cement should be used for lining. Extra thickness of composite can be added buccally if this is a problem with the finished restoration

7 Comprehensive Care: Examples of Treated Cases

The aim of this chapter is to illustrate some clinical cases requiring comprehensive paediatric dental treatment. It should never be forgotten when planning treatment that children are not 'miniature adults', and each child has a different personality, anxieties and dental treatment needs. The treatment plan should therefore be tailor-made for each child, with the aim being not just to treat the dentition but also to instil a positive dental attitude. Therefore the principles of assessment and treatment planning, as discussed in Chapter 1, are of paramount importance and have been used to illustrate the cases shown here.

Each case is presented with full pre- and post-operative clinical photographs and radiographs, including recall visit radiographs taken for a minimum period of one year post-operatively. Accompanying each case is a brief history, a full treatment plan by visit, including assessment and introduction to dentistry, preventive programme and the restorative treatment. The preventive programme included oral hygiene assessment, dietary analysis, caries susceptibility tests, fissure sealants and the use of fluorides. Space mainte-

nance was carried out where necessary. All three comprehensive cases presented illustrate the use of advanced paediatric dental techniques, described in the preceding chapters.

In our opinion, every child deserves the standard of care illustrated in this chapter.

CASE A

The following case is an example of advanced restorative procedures in a pre-school child.

Background

Past dental history

'John' was a 3½-year-old boy who had previously attended a dentist, with little restorative work having been carried out. There was a history of pain from several teeth, but no specific tooth could be identified as causing symptoms.

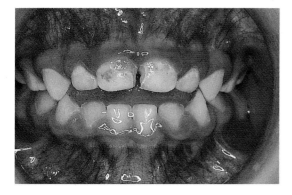

Figure 7.1 Anterior view showing mesio-buccal caries 51 and 61, buccal caries in 62 and demineralization on the buccal surfaces of 52, 53, and 63.

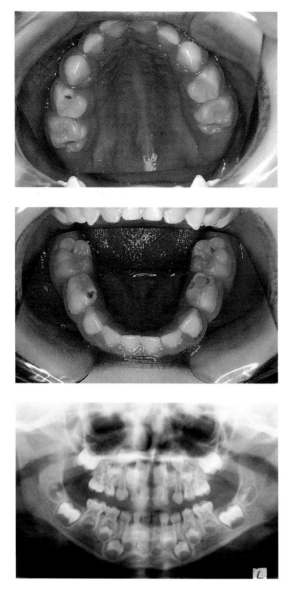

Figure 7.2 Upper occlusal view showing caries in the occlusal surfaces of 54, 55, 64 and 65.

Figure 7.3 Lower occlusal view showing occlusal caries in 75, 84 and 85 and a failed glass ionomer cement restoration in 74. There was also distal caries in 83. A further finding was a small enamel pearl on the occlusal surface of 85.

Figure 7.4 Orthopantomogram showing caries in 55, 54, 51, 61, 64, 65, 75, 74, 84 and 85. The radiograph also shows pulpal involvement of 74.

Past medical history

There were no medical complications relevant to dental treatment.

Intra-oral findings

Extensive decay was found in several of the primary molars and also in the upper central incisors, as can be seen in Figures 7.1–7.3.

Radiographic assessment

An orthopantomogram radiograph was taken (Figure 7.4), which shows the extent of the caries in the primary molars. At this stage John's cooperation was not sufficient to allow intra-oral radiographs.

Behaviour assessment

John was rated as being moderately apprehensive but cooperative. An introductory visit was necessary to familiarize him with the clinical environment and with the equipment that would be used. A mixture of 'tell–show–do' and behaviour shaping was planned to give a step-by-step introduction of hand and rotary instruments, topical and local analgesia, rubber dam and restorative treatment.

Preventive assessment

John's high caries level meant that prevention would be an important part of the treatment plan. This would need to include diet analysis, oral hygiene, fluoride supplementation and progress monitored with the use of caries susceptibility tests (*S. Mutans* counts).

Treatment plan

A treatment plan was drawn up as follows.

Visit 1 (initial visit)

- Examination, radiographs, prophylaxis; outline treatment plan
- Diet history sheet given
- Initial caries susceptibility test carried out
- Treatment and preventive plan discussed with parents

Visit 2

- Introduction to surgery and techniques
- Dressing of open cavities with intermediate restorative material (IRM)
- Prophylaxis
- Collection of diet history sheet
- Results of caries tests
- Fluoride supplements prescribed
-

Visit 3

- Local analgesia and rubber dam
- 64 occlusal composite resin
- 65 occlusal composite resin
- Fluoride varnish (Duraphat) placed on demineralized areas
- Discussion of diet analysis

Visit 4

- Local analgesia and rubber dam
- 55 occlusal composite resin
- 54 occlusal composite resin
- Recheck oral hygiene

Visit 5

- Local analgesia and rubber dam
- 75 occlusal amalgam
- 74 pulp treatment and SSC

Visit 6

- Local analgesia and rubber dam
- 83 composite resin
- 84 pulp treatment and SSC
- 85 occlusal composite resin
- Retest caries susceptibility
- Reinforce prevention programme

Visit 7

- Local analgesia and rubber dam
- 51 strip crown
- 61 strip crown
- 62 buccal composite resin

- Polish restorations
- Reinforce preventive advice
- Arrange 4-month recall appointment

The postoperative intra-oral photographs and radiographs are shown in Figures 7.5–7.10.

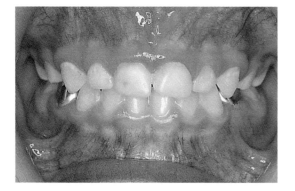

Figure 7.5 Anterior view showing strip crowns on 51 and 61 and the composite in 62. It can also be noted that there is no deterioration of the demineralized areas.

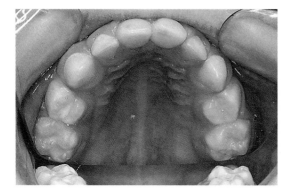

Figure 7.6 Upper occlusal view showing composite resins placed in 55, 54, 64, and 65. It also shows an incisal view of the strip crowns on 51 and 61.

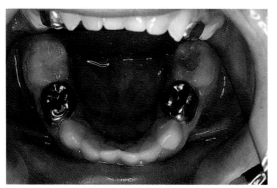

Figure 7.7 Lower occlusal view showing SSC on 74 and 84, amalgam restoration in 75 and composite resin restoration in 85.

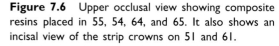

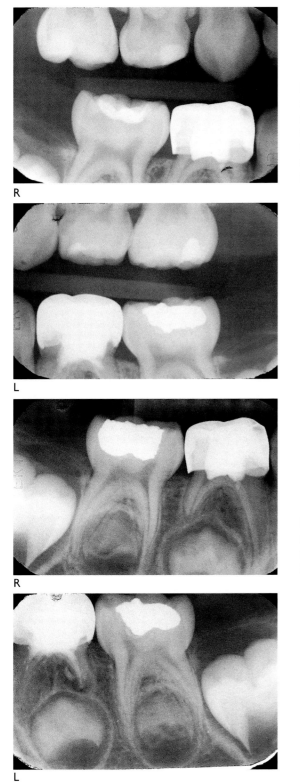

R

L

R

L

Figure 7.8 Follow-up bitewing radiographs four months post-operatively showing normal furcation areas on 74 and 84. Recurrent caries was noted around the enamel pearl on 85, which extended under the composite restoration. This restoration was therefore removed together with the caries and replaced with amalgam.

Figure 7.9 Peri-apical radiographs six months post-operatively showing no deterioration in the furcation areas of 74 and 84. The restoration in 85, which was replaced with amalgam, can also be seen.

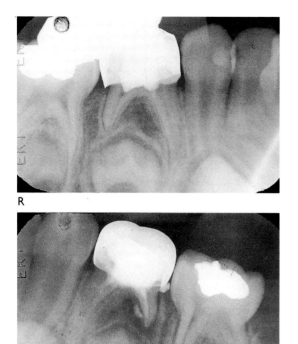

R

L

Figure 7.10 Peri-apical radiographs one year post-operatively showing no deterioration in the furcation areas.

CASE B

The following case is an example of advanced restorative procedures in a 6-year-old child.

Background

Past dental history

'Jasmine' was a 6-year-old girl with limited past dental experience and a history of poor dental attendance. She presented with extensive dental caries, but no history of dental pain.

Past medical history

There were no medical complications relevant to dental treatment.

Intra-oral findings

Figures 7.11–7.13 show the intra-oral findings pre-treatment. Dental caries was evident in 55, 54, 61, 64 (roots), 65, 75, 84 and 85.

Radiographs

An orthopantomogram (Figure 7.14) and bitewing radiographs (Figure 7.15) were taken, and showed complete development of the permanent dentition. The first permanent molars were erupting. Caries involved a number of primary teeth, but there did not appear to be any pulpal involvement or any peri-apical pathology.

Behaviour assessment

Jasmine was rated apprehensive but cooperative, or +/– using the Wright–Frankl scale. An introductory

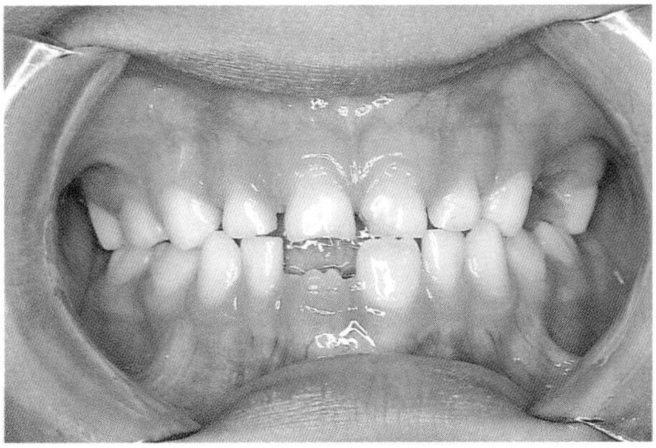

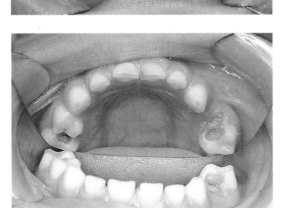

Figure 7.11 Anterior view showing mesial caries in 61 and 65 and broken down 64.

Figure 7.12 Upper occlusal view showing caries in 55, 54, 61 and 65, and the root remnants of 64.

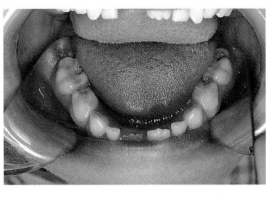

Figure 7.13   Lower occlusal view showing caries in 75, 74, 84 and 85.

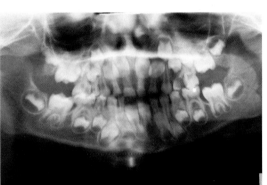

Figure 7.14   Orthopantomogram showing caries in 55, 54, 61, 64 (roots), 65, 75, 74, 84 and 85.

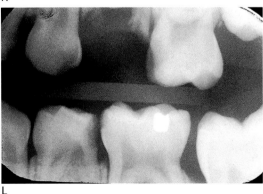
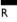

Figure 7.15   Bitewing radiographs showing caries in 55, 54, 64 (roots), 65, 75, 74, 84 and 85.

visit was planned to introduce her to dentistry and in particular the use of rotary instruments. The use of TSD was planned to introduce the use of hand and rotary instruments, together with the use of local analgesia.

Preventive assessment

Because of the high level of dental caries, a preventive programme was included in the treatment plan. This required a review of oral hygiene, dietary analysis and the use of fluoride as part of the preventive programme. The role of prevention was discussed with the parents and its importance stressed. The first permanent molars were in the process of erupting, and therefore fissure sealants would be needed during the course of treatment or at a recall visit.

Treatment plan

A treatment plan was drawn up as follows.

Visit I (initial visit)

- Examination, radiographs, oral hygiene assessment, prophylaxis, outline of treatment plan
- Diet history sheet given
- Caries susceptibility test (*S. mutans* counts)
- Application of fluoride varnish
- Treatment and preventive plan discussed with parents

Visit 2

- Introduction to surgery and techniques
- Dressing of open cavities with IRM
- Oral hygiene assessment and prophylaxis
- Collection of diet history sheet
- Results of caries tests
- Daily fluoride mouthrinse prescribed

Visit 3

- Local analgesia and rubber dam
- 65 remove caries and place SSC
- 64 extraction of roots
- Impressions for study models
- Discussion about diet

Visit 4

- Local analgesia and rubber dam
- 55 remove caries and place SSC
- 54 remove caries and place SSC
- Recheck oral hygiene
- Space analysis

Visit 5

- Local analgesia and rubber dam
- 75 remove caries and place SSC
- 74 remove caries and place SSC

Visit 6

- Local analgesia and rubber dam
- 85 remove caries and place SSC
- 84 remove caries and place SSC
- Retest caries susceptibility
- Reinforce prevention programme
- Band fitted 65 and impression for band and loop space maintainer

Visit 7

- Fit band and loop space maintainer
- Fissure-seal 36 and 46
- Polish restorations
- Reinforce preventive advice
- Arrange 4-month recall appointment (fissure-seal 16 and 26 on eruption)

The post-operative photographs and radiographs are shown in Figures 7.16–7.20.

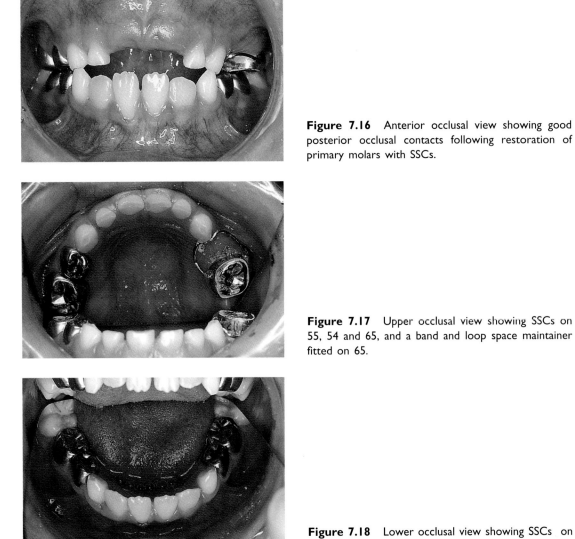

Figure 7.16 Anterior occlusal view showing good posterior occlusal contacts following restoration of primary molars with SSCs.

Figure 7.17 Upper occlusal view showing SSCs on 55, 54 and 65, and a band and loop space maintainer fitted on 65.

Figure 7.18 Lower occlusal view showing SSCs on 75, 74, 84 and 85, and fissure sealants on 36 and 46.

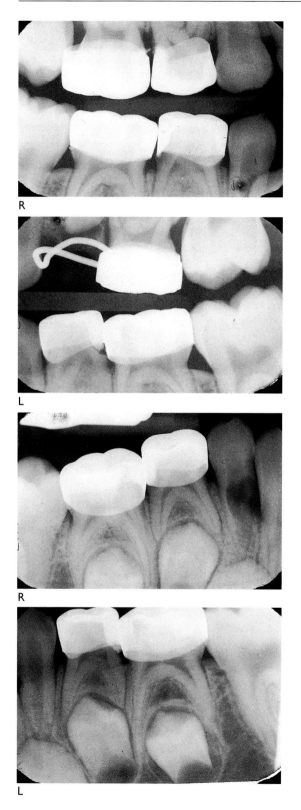

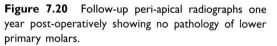

Figure 7.19 Follow-up bitewing radiographs four months post-operatively showing no evidence of dental caries.

Figure 7.20 Follow-up peri-apical radiographs one year post-operatively showing no pathology of lower primary molars.

CASE C

The following case is an example of multiple pulp therapies in a 5-year-old child.

Background

Past dental history

'Robert' was a 5-year-old boy with a history of irregular attendance. The cavities that had been noted several months previously had now become more extensive, and were causing pain with cold and sweet foods. Some small restorations had been attempted in the past.

Past medical history

The only medical complications relevant to Robert's dental treatment were that he was allergic to penicillin and that he was slightly deaf.

Intra-oral findings

Figures 7.21–7.23 show the intra-oral findings. There was extensive caries affecting all primary molars and very early lesions on the upper central incisors. No tooth was tender to percussion, and there was no abscess or draining sinus.

Radiographic assessment

Initial radiographic assessment included an orthopantomogram and a peri-apical view to assess possible peri-apical and furcation involvement of 75 (Figures 7.24 and 7.25).

Behaviour assessment

Robert was considered to be fairly cooperative but a little slow at comprehending instructions. It was decided that behaviour management should include the 'tell–show–do' technique in a form compatible with Robert's understanding, using step-by-step instructions and demonstrations. It was also important to assess the motivation of the family towards dental treatment before embarking on a long and complicated treatment plan.

Preventive assessment

As with cases A and B, Robert had high caries levels, so prevention was a high priority. As before, this would include oral hygiene, diet analysis, fluoride supplements and caries susceptibility testing.

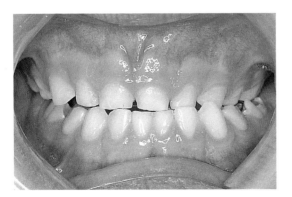

Figure 7.21 Anterior view showing early lesions in 51 and 61 and an idea of the extent of some of the posterior cavities, together with the resulting loss in occlusal height.

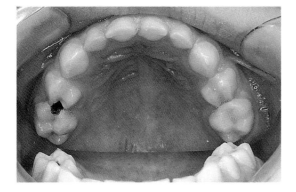

Figure 7.22 Upper occlusal view showing carious lesions in 54 and 55 affecting the marginal ridges of both teeth. Also shadowing on the occlusal surfaces of 64 and 65 suggests lesions within these teeth too.

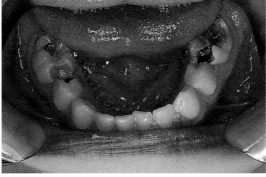

Figure 7.23 Lower occlusal view showing marginal ridge involvement of 74 and 84, and very extensive lesions in both 75 and 85.

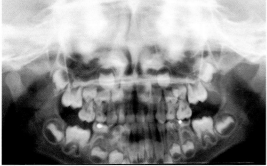

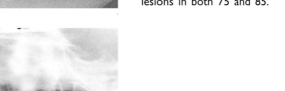

Figure 7.24 Orthopantomogram confirming carious involvement of 55, 54, 64, 65, 75, 74, 84 and 85. It should also be noted that the first permanent molars were near to eruption and that there was the possibility that 16 might erupt ectopically.

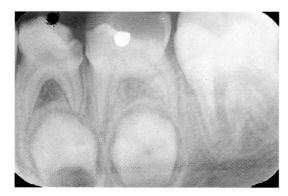

Figure 7.25 Péri-apical radiograph of 75 and 74 showing no furcation involvement.

Treatment plan

A treatment plan was drawn up as follows.

Visit 1

- Examination, radiographs
- Oral hygiene assessment, prophylaxis
- Diet history sheet given
- Caries susceptibility test carried out
- Treatment and preventive plan discussed with parents

Visit 2

- Introduction
- Dressing of open cavities with IRM
- Prophylaxis
- Collection of diet history sheet
- Results of caries tests
- Fluoride supplements prescribed

Visit 3

- Local analgesia and rubber dam
- 64 remove caries and place SSC
- 65 remove caries and place SSC
- Discussion of diet analysis
- Duraphat varnish on early lesions 51 and 61

Visit 4

- Local analgesia and rubber dam
- 54 pulpotomy and SSC
- 55 pulpotomy and SSC
- Recheck oral hygiene

Visit 5

- Local analgesia and rubber dam
- 75 pulpotomy and SSC
- 74 pulpotomy and SSC
- Check use of fluoride supplements
- Duraphat on 51 and 61

Visit 6

- Local analgesia and rubber dam
- 84 pulpotomy and SSC
- 85 pulpotomy and SSC
- Retest caries susceptibility

Visit 7

- Check all restorations
- Reinforce oral hygiene and prevention programme
- Results of caries tests
- Arrange 3-month recall, with the plan to fissure-seal first permanent molars on eruption

The post-operative intra-oral photographs and radiographs are shown in Figures 7.26–7.30.

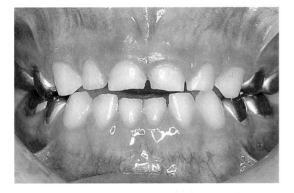

Figure 7.26 Anterior view showing improvement of occlusion following placement of stainless steel crowns. There has also been no deterioration of the early lesions in 51 and 61.

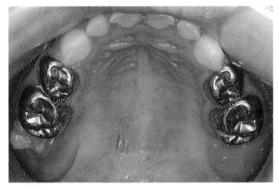

Figure 7.27 Upper occlusal view showing stainless steel crowns on all upper primary molars.

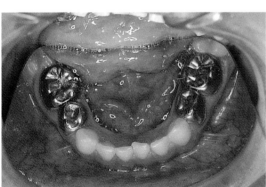

Figures 7.28 Lower occlusal view showing stainless steel crowns placed on all lower primary molars.

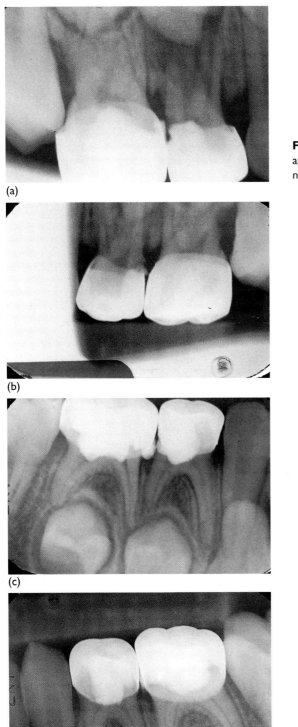

(a)

(b)

(c)

(d)

Figure 7.29 (a–d) Four-months post-operative peri-apical radiographs of the primary molars showing normal peri-apical and furcation areas.

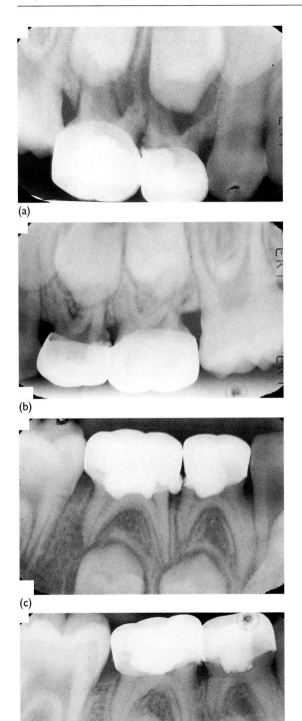

(a)

(b)

(c)

(d)

Figure 7.30 (a–d) One-year post-operative peri-apical radiographs of the primary molars showing no change in the furcation areas.

Further Reading

Local analgesia

Adatia AK, Regional nerve block for maxillary permanent molars, *Br Dent J* (1976) **140**:87–92.

Roberts DH, Sowray JH, *Local analgesia in dentistry*, 3rd edn (John Wright: Bristol 1987).

Rubber dam

Cochran MA, Miller CH, Sheldrake MA, The efficacy of rubber dam as a barrier to the spread of microorganisms during dental treatment, *J Am Dent Assoc* (1989) **119**:141–4.

Gergely EJ, Desmond Greer Walker Award. Rubber dam acceptance, *Br Dent J* (1989) **167**:249–52.

Jones CM, Reid J, Patient and operator attitudes towards rubber dam, *J Dent Child* (1988) **55**:452–4.

Marshall K, Page J, The use of rubber dam in the UK: a survey, *Br Dent J* (1990) **169**:286–91.

The pulpotomy technique

Doyle WA, McDonald RE, Mitchell DF, Formocresol versus calcium hydroxide in pulpotomy, *J Dent Child* (1962) **29**:86–97.

Feigal RJ, Messer HH, A critical look at gluteraldehyde, *Pediatr Dent* (1990) **12**:69–71.

Fei A, Udin R, Johnson R, A clinical study of ferric sulfate as a pulpotomy agent in 10 teeth, *Pediatr Dent* (1991) **13**:327–32.

Fuks AB, Bimstein E, A clinical evaluation of diluted formocresol pulpotomies in primary teeth of school children, *Pediatr Dent* (1981) **3**:321–4.

Fuks A, Michael Y, Sofer-Saks B et al, Enriched collagen solution as a pulp dressing in pulpotomized teeth in monkeys, *Pediatr Dent* (1984) **6**:243–7.

Garcia-Godoy F, A 42 month clinical evaluation of gluteraldehyde pulpotomies in primary teeth, *J Pedod* (1986) **10**:148–55.

s'Gravenmade EJ, Some biochemical considerations on fixation in endodontics, *J Endodon* (1975) **1**:233–7.

Hobson P, Pulp treatment of deciduous teeth: II. Clinical investigation, *Br Dent J* (1970) **128**:232–8.

Ketley CE, Goodman JR, Formocresol toxicity: is there a suitable alternative for pulpotomy of primary molars? *Int J Paediatr Dent* (1990) **2**:12–15.

Lazzari EP, Ranly D, Walker WA, Biochemical effects of formocresol on bovine pulp tissue, *Oral Surg* (1978) **45**:796–802.

Magnusson B, Therapeutic pulpotomies in primary molars with formocresol technique, *Acta Odont Scand* (1978) **36**:157–65.

Morawa AP, Straffon LH, Han SS, Clinical evaluation of pulpotomies using dilute formocresol, *J Dent Child* (1975) **42**: 360–3.

Mudler GR, Van Amerongen WE, Vingerling PA, Consequences of endodontic treatment of primary teeth. II. A clinical investigation into the influence of formocresol pulpotomy on the permanent successor, *J Dent Child* (1987) **54**:35–9.

Myers DR, Pashley DH, Tissue changes induced by absorption of formocresol from pulpotomy sites in dogs, *Pediatr Dent* (1983) **5**:6–8.

Pruhs RJ, Olen GA, Sharma PS, Relationship between formocresol pulpotomy in primary teeth and enamel defects in their permanent successors, *J Am Dent Assoc* (1977) **94**:698–700.

Roolling I, Hasselgren G, Tronstad L, Morphological and enzyme histochemical observations on the pulp of human primary molars 3 to 5 years after formocresol treatment, *Oral Surg* (1976) **42**:58–28.

Roolling I, Lambjerg-Hansen H, Pulp conditions of successfully treated primary molars, *Scand J Dent Res* (1978) **86**:267–72.

Roolling I, Poulsen S, Formocresol pulpotomy of primary teeth and occurance of enamel defects on permanent successors, *Acta Odontol Scand* (1978) **36**:243–7.

Schroder U, A 2 year follow-up of 10 molars pulpotomized with a gentle technique and capped with calcium hydroxide, *Scand J Dent Res* (1978) **86**:273–8.

Shaw BW, Sheller B, Barrus BD et al, Electrosurgical pulpotomy—a six month study in primates, *J Endod* (1987) **13**:500–5.

Shoji S, Hariuchi H et al, Histopathological changes in dental pulp irradiated with CO_2 laser: a preliminary report on laser pulpotomy, *J Endod* (1985) **11**:379–84.

Wright FA, Widmer RP, Pulp therapy in primary teeth: a retrospective study, *J Pedod* (1979) **3**:195–206.

The pulpectomy technique

Aylard SR, Johnson R, Assessment of filling techniques for primary teeth, *Pediatr Dent* (1987) **9**:195–8.

Barr ES, Flaitz CM, Hicks MJ, A retrospective radiographic evaluation of primary molar pulpectomies, *Pediatr Dent* (1991) **13**:4–8.

Coll JA, Casper JS, Evaluation of one appointment formocresol pulpectomy technique for primary molars, *Pediatr Dent* (1988) **10**:178–84.

Duggal MS, Curzon MEJ, Restoration of the broken down primary molar: I. Pulpectomy technique, *Dental Update* (1989) **16**:26–8.

Garcia-Godoy F, Evaluation of an iodoform paste in root canal therapy for infected primary teeth, *J Dent Child* (1987) **54**:30–4.

Gould JM, Root canal therapy for infected primary molar teeth: preliminary report, *J Dent Child* (1972) **29**:269–73.

McDonald RE, Avery DR, *Dentistry for the child and adolescent*, 5th edn (Mosby: St Louis 1988) 435–65.

Paterson SA, Curzon MEJ, The effect of amoxycillin versus penicillin V in the treatment of acutely abscessed primary teeth, *Br Dent J* (1993) **174**:443–9.

Stainless steel crowns for primary molars

Braff MA, A comparison between stainless steel crowns and multisurface amalgams in primary molars, *J Dent Child* (1975) **42**:474–8.

Dawson LT, Simon JR, Taylor PP, The use of amalgam and stainless steel crown restorations for primary molars, *J Dent Child* (1981) **48**:420–2.

Duggal MS, Curzon MEJ, Restoration of the broken down primary molar: 2. Stainless steel crowns, *Dental Update* (1989) **16**:71–5.

McDonald RE, Avery DR, *Dentistry for the child and adolescent*, 5th edn (Mosby: St Louis 1988) 403–34.

O'Sullivan E, Curzon MEJ, The efficacy of comprehensive dental care for children under general anaesthesia, *Br Dent J* (1991) **171**:56–8.

Roberts JF, Sharif M, The fate and survival of amalgams and preformed crown molar restorations placed in specialist paediatric dental practice, *Br Dent J* (1990) **169**:237–44.

Strip crowns for primary incisors

Doyle WA, A new preparation for primary incisor jackets, *Pediatr Dent* (1979) **1**:38–40.

Kennedy DB, *Operative paediatric dentistry* (John Wright: Bristol 1986).

Pollard MA, Curzon JA, Fenlon WL, The restoration of decayed primary incisors using strip crowns, *Dental Update* (1991) **18**:150–2.

Weinberger SJ, Treatment modalities for primary incisors, *Canadian Dent Assoc J* (1989) **55**:807–2.

Index